The Modern

Rapunzel

Who is Rapunzel?

She is known as the fairytale princess held captive in a tower by an evil enchantress. During the time of her imprisonment, Rapunzel grew long golden tresses resembling spun gold. Her hair was so strong and thick that her Prince was able to climb "the golden stair" to rescue her.

Rapunzel is one of my favorite fairytale characters. When the story was read to me as a child, I envisioned having long, luscious golden hair of my own strong enough for my prince to climb if I ever got trapped in a tower and needed to be rescued.

Why is the story of Rapunzel now fitting in this day and age besides being a reminder of one of childhood's delights? Why is this book called *The Modern Rapunzel*?

Like the original Rapunzel, the modern Rapunzel has been captive. Instead of being held captive in a tower, the modern Rapunzel is held back by the mysteries of how to have the hair of her dreams and live her beauty.

How did Rapunzel grow such beautiful, long and thick hair strong enough for her prince to climb? What were her secrets? They were never revealed!

Finally, here is the back story of her secrets, for the woman of today.

Like the fairytale Rapunzel, the modern Rapunzel has been rescued. With this book, she now has the knowledge she needs to fulfill her wishes. You can make your own fairytale come true.

Who is the modern Rapunzel?

The Modern Rapunzel is you.

The Modern Rapunzel

Natural Secrets for Ending Hair Loss (and Other Miracles)

Jeanne Powers

DISCLAIMER

I have been involved in self-study for over 40 years. The information you are about to read is based on my own research and application of what I have learned. I have consistently applied the techniques presented in this book, which, without fail, have worked for me. Every person is unique. Some of these procedures may work for you, some may not. There is no promise of a cure.

Sprinkled throughout this book I've placed inspirational quotes for your enjoyment. I assume no responsibility for all the fun you'll have while reading the stories and information.

I am required to say that everything in this book is my opinion and if you do anything I recommend without the advice or supervision of a licensed medical doctor or cosmetologist, you do so at your own risk. The information contained in this book is not intended to serve as medical advice, nor should it be used for diagnosing or treating a health problem or disease. The author presents this information for educational purposes only. There is no attempt to prescribe any medical treatment and if you are ill or suspect you may have a health problem, it is recommended you seek the advice of a competent, licensed health-care provider.

The author assumes no responsibility for errors, omissions, or contrary interpretations of the subject matter herein.

No warranties, expressed or implied, are offered with any information, services or products presented in this book.

Jeanne Powers

ISBN: 978-1477601051

Printed in USA

Book design by Alan Gilbertson, G&G Creative, Los Angeles

Contents

Part One

How to Create a Beautiful Head of Hair

Part Two

You: The Whole Woman

Appendices

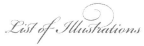

List of Illustrations

The Licensed Material is being used for illustrative purposes only and any person depicted in the Licensed Material is a model.

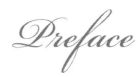

Preface

You are about to experience a breakthrough in having the hair of your dreams. If you have longed for thick, gorgeous hair, you are in the right place at the right time.

Many years ago I lost over half my head of hair. My shower drain was clogged with an alarming amount of fallen hair and my brush looked like a little matted wig. I was panicked to put it mildly.

For an extended period of time prior to that, my hair was lifeless, thin and wouldn't grow. I wondered what was wrong that I couldn't grow a thick, beautiful head of hair.

I took it upon myself to find the answers. I refused to go the toxic chemical "cure" route.

What makes this book unique is that I lived through the nightmares of hair loss, thin, unhealthy and damaged hair myself. I came through it shining, having gained the knowledge, experience and results I'm now passing on to you.

I wish I would have had this book when I so desperately needed it.

If you want to know—as I did...

- ❧ why hair falls out and how to turn it around,
- ❧ the proven essential tools of what to do to help handle a hair crisis *today*,
- ❧ simple actions to take that will help make your hair thicker, stronger, shinier, healthier and more beautiful and keep it that way for a lifetime,
- ❧ proven and practical action steps for hair problems without having to sort through technical terminology to get the needed information and understanding,
- ❧ how to naturally improve the condition of your hair and scalp without resorting to drugs, surgery and toxic chemically-based

products which challenge and ultimately defeat the healing laws of Mother Nature,

and in the process...

❧ learn the basics on how to look and feel more youthful and energetic,

...then you are about to read such a book.

A great deal of this information is new. The discoveries are a result of personal, sometimes very challenging experiences of one woman's journey to beauty and health.

This hard-won knowledge provides the answers on how to stop hair loss, grow your hair back, have gorgeous locks and bring out your own radiance, naturally. It also incorporates successful key lifestyle elements for optimum overall health and happiness.

Women have poured out their hearts to me on how their thin or thinning hair affects the way they feel about themselves and how it has stopped or slowed them down from reaching out in life the way they want.

Upon implementing the procedures in this book, these women have written success stories sharing how thrilled they are with the results and how their lives have changed. I am just, if not more, thrilled than they are.

After years of frustration, they have reported they are growing in new hair and that their hair has become thicker, stronger and growing at an accelerated rate. Those who had "tired," dry or lifeless hair, now have locks they can call their Crowning Glory. Some of these success stories are at the end of this book and on my website www.themodernrapunzel.com.

I've also received wonderful success stories from readers who have smoother, softer skin and have reduced or eliminated wrinkles as a result of applying the simple, natural skin procedures in Appendix 1.

As stress is a key reason for hair-loss I've devoted an entire chapter to this subject and how to handle its effects in daily living. After reading Chapter 13, "The Factors of Stress and Hair Loss" and Part Two, "You, The Whole Woman," readers have shared their life-changing shifts of viewpoint regarding beauty, stress and "aging." This provides relief, inspiration, and dramatically increases self-confidence.

We know a hair crisis isn't fun. At the beginning of Chapter Two is a three-step process called "The Magic Overnight Hair Beautification

Procedure." It's the proven method of what to do now to help handle a current hair crisis. Once you've implemented these three simple steps you'll see your existing hair has more beauty, fullness and strength.

This procedure does more for hair as an instant and long-term handling for dryness and for damage than anything I've ever seen or personally experienced, all accomplished naturally. Many women have said these three steps, all on their own, have given them the results they were looking for.

If your hair is thin or noticeably thinning, once you apply "The Magic Overnight Hair Beautification Procedure," you'll see each existing hair will have more fullness. It will then be easier to carry out the hair-growth procedures as outlined in the book as there's less or little attention on the current appearance of your hair.

Once implemented, you also won't feel the need to resort to potentially damaging solutions in the attempt to make your hair look fuller now, such as a perm or other unnatural solutions. This is important as these desperate solutions can result in more hair loss.

There are also individual sections in the book on how to grow long hair, create shine and prevent breakage, help handle dandruff naturally, itchy scalp, dryness and graying.

To make it easier for you, there are charts in the back for an at-a-glance look at what to do according to the condition of your hair from: "Needs a Little Help," to "I'm Starting to Get Worried," to "Yikes! My Hair, What There Is Left of It, Is a Disaster!" You now have immediate access to the program designed for the category of your hair.

While implementing the basic steps as outlined in the charts, you'll find it beneficial and rewarding to refer back to relevant sections in the book as many times as needed until you have complete clarity on what to do. You'll find many details you may have missed, details which the charts themselves cannot provide. Please read the whole book first and then use the charts as your overall guide.

For those of you in the category of "I'm Starting to Get Worried" or "Yikes! My Hair, What There Is Left of It, Is a Disaster!," I recommend reading "The Factors of Stress and Hair Loss" first. Stress takes the #1 toll on the body. Getting on top of stress is essential in preventing hair loss and ensuring a new growth of hair. Successful management of stressful elements in one's life is a must in any healing process. Reading this section first will help provide relief and inspiration so the hair procedures can then take hold. A body will repair and rejunvenate when given the chance.

I've had many readers ask where to get high-quality natural shampoos, conditioners and other products. On my website, www.themodernrapunzel.com is a Products section with the information on where to obtain them.

While reading, you may have questions. More than likely they will be addressed later on in the book. Those that aren't, email your question(s) to jeanne@themodernrapunzel.com and put in the subject line "Question on hair." I am happy to then answer you in a newsletter or blog which you will receive monthly. Some of the answers may require research, so be patient.

Now that I have created thick, beautiful hair and have learned the keys to health and beauty and a more youthful appearance, it is truly my joy to provide you with this life-changing information.

Through the secrets you're about to discover combined with your care, love and nurturing, you can create the head of hair you've always wanted!

You're about to embark on an exciting and fulfilling journey.

Let's begin!

Acknowledgments

Through inspiration and support from loved ones a book comes to fruition. Without Magnificent family and friends this book would have never happened.

I would like to acknowledge:

- Ron, who spent his whole life bringing out the beauty in others and who is my never-ending inspiration,
- my Mother who has always unfailingly supported my dreams,
- Scott, the love of my life who brings out the natural woman and artist in me,
- Jack and Kelly, whose mentoring made this project pure joy,
- Annie and Rivka who taught me what it is to be a woman,
- Bernard and Merry who have been my spiritual catalysts and who, without them, this book would have sat on the shelf until I was 90,
- Pam, my staunchest supporter and always there for me with every detail,
- Helyn, my dear Cosmetologist friend who has been the last word on technical advice and who has unfailingly given me support throughout this whole project,
- Jessie, my Illustrator, who put her heart into bringing the concepts to life,
- Linda, Margo and Helyn, my Editors, who ensured everything makes complete sense,
- Debbie, Lee, Marie and Kevin who have always been there for me for anything I've needed,
- and a very special acknowledgement, Alan-Worth-His-Weight-In-Gold-Gilbertson, my creative director, book designer and inspirational guide who has gone way above and beyond all

expectations in every aspect of this project. His flawless pro-
fessionalism and exceptional knowledge created challenges
for me and through his insistence on perfection, pushed me
further than I ever thought I could go. He was always right.
You have all been the beacon of light bringing life to my big dreams.
Thank you, Dear Ones.

Introduction

The information you are about to read is simple, basic and practical. It has been researched and developed with loving and diligent care over a period of many years.

Throughout the process of discovering genuine solutions, I read, experimented, sorted, sifted and applied what worked and threw out what didn't. I kept my "antennae" alert for information that would create a beautiful head of hair, true health and beauty.

I ran to my desk well over a hundred times to give myself reminders of what should be included in this book.

Why has this been so important to me? Because I know what it was like to have had my attention riveted on the way my hair looked and the way I felt. I was introverted and unhappy to a very large degree.

Perhaps it's not that bad for you but if it is, know I understand completely.

My purpose for writing this book is to provide women with natural, safe and effective solutions for the problems we face with our hair. As hair is so intimate to us and affects our sense of well-being so strongly, if I am able to, in any way, help you remove the barriers to being able to shine as the unique and special individual you are, I will have done my job. I feel it is vital we are able to freely express ourselves in life according to our own desires without the distraction of wishing we looked differently.

This book encompasses the whole picture of beautiful hair, physical health and you. Each one of these three factors can positively or negatively affect the others. All of them, individually and together, are indicators of how we look and feel.

There are many influencing factors regarding hair loss. By reading the information contained in this book you will be availing yourself of the complete range of knowledge, understanding and tools for healthy hair for a lifetime.

This is not a technical manual filled with "whys and wherefores" or terminology which inevitably leads off into other tangents of study. My intention is to provide you with the information that appeals to your common sense so you can think for yourself.

Perhaps I will replace some solutions you have that may not be proving successful even though you've maintained hope they might work. Perhaps I will remind you of what you "forgot" and only need to be reminded of. Some of what I say you've heard before. That's because it works. Most of it will be new to you.

There is a great deal of information here, but it is simple, understandable and very do-able. There is no need to be overwhelmed. Take your time. Find one or two actions you can do something about now, implement them and then return to the book and charts for the next actions to take.

At nineteen, I had a wake-up call when I discovered "authorities" didn't have the answers I was personally seeking. I will share that story and others. I will hold nothing back. Even though you don't know me, I hope by the time you finish this book, you will.

Friends tell me I look fifteen or more years younger than I am. I have a thick, healthy mane of gorgeous hair and smooth skin with a small number of minor wrinkles on my face. I'm not bragging. It's the truth. It's not through good fortune, leading a pampered life, expensive creams, drugs, taking a million supplements, or living off tofu or grapes. I'm not a successful actress or model with the financial wherewithal for plastic surgery, nor have I ever resorted to the newest drug that grows hair or the latest expensive skin products that do this or that.

The truth is I never desired to go that route as I chose to follow a simple, instinctive one.

I started the process over 40 years ago when my hair was thin, wouldn't grow and had little shine. At one point I lost over half of my head of hair. Since then I have found the answers that have proven successful; those that have withstood the test of time. This book is a compilation of those procedures taken to grow the head of hair I now have.

The short and long-term solutions I've used on my own hair are tried-and-true. Once in a while I add to them but I never change what has worked.

For many years I haven't had to be as diligent as I was when my hair was originally in bad shape. Initially you will need to set your mind to applying the procedures and routines until you have the head of hair you want. Then, it's just maintenance.

In this day and age we are flooded with information and products. How do we rise to the task of identifying the essentials that not only make sense but are health-giving and actually work?

I feel I will have accomplished a great deal if I have saved you years of trial and error in the search for answers and natural, safe and effective solutions.

One of my other hopes is that I can assist you in refraining from potentially damaging solutions, solutions that could be resorted to out of a desperate need to do something now! Thus, The Magic Overnight Hair Beautification Procedure was born.

Along with having thin and lifeless hair those many years ago, I dealt with very sensitive skin and was allergic to polluted environments. Being chemically sensitive, it was a continuous struggle to look and feel good. I had to come up with natural remedies because I demanded to look and feel the way I wanted. I was sensitive to everything around me and still am which is why I have written this book, providing what I discovered. Now I know being "sensitive" has served to my advantage.

When I started this process I insisted on having a luscious head of hair and defy aging. Wanting to look great is not vain. It is natural.

Having a glorious head of hair and looking and feeling 15-20 years younger than I am makes me very happy. I want you to be happy with the way you look, too.

Let's create some hair magic!

How to Create a

Beautiful

Head of Hair

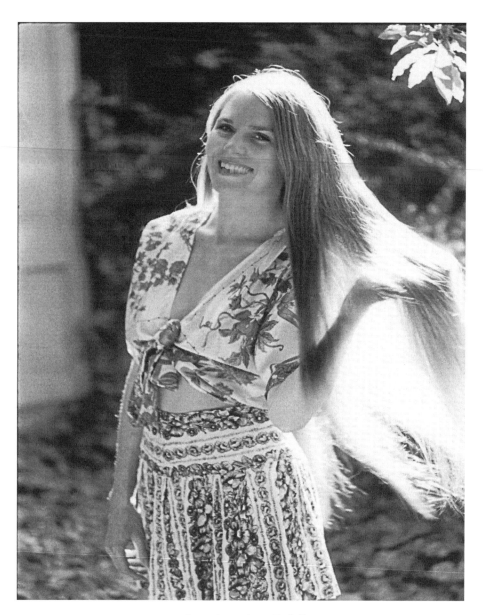

1975 – Los Angeles, California

Chapter One

Hair —
a Woman's Crowning Glory!

*"Women...Who made 'em? God must have been a...genius.
Their hair. They say that the hair is everything, you know?
Have you ever buried your nose in a mountain of curls, and
just wanted to go to sleep forever?"*

**Bo Goldman "The Start of an Education"
made popular by the movie Scent of a Woman.**

In the 60's, during the era of the Flower Children, my hair was everything (and still is). I longed to have a man bury his nose in my hair, happy to go to sleep forever in my abundant, lush locks! But, my hair was lifeless, thin and wouldn't grow past the top of my shoulders. I was most unhappy about it. My two best friends had beautiful hair down to their waists. Waist-length, flowing hair was definitely "in."

I started researching everything I could get my hands on, went to a seminar given by a famous authority on hair, tried pulling my hair to make it longer (just kidding), and so on and so on. Call it an obsession. That's okay. I was determined. I figured if I wanted something bad enough, I'd get it. I was right.

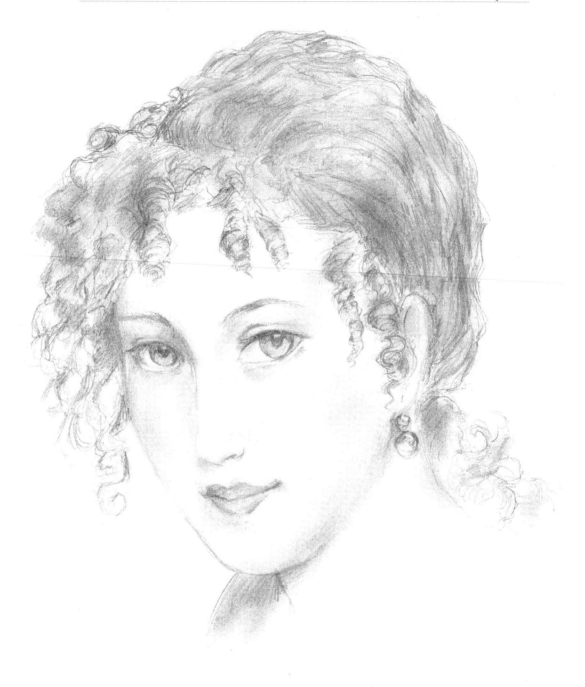

"The hair is the richest ornament of women."
Martin Luther

It actually started when I was a senior in high school. I still can't believe my teacher let me get away with it, but he did. I sat in the front row of my history class for several days each month and pulled each little section of hair around in front of my eyes, bit by bit, so I could see it. And then hair-by-hair I checked for split ends, making very sure I cut only those ends that were split. I did this because I had learned that split ends prevent the hair from getting long. Besides, split ends just weren't cool!

So now you should have a pretty good idea how determined (and you may think crazy) I was. I was a hopeful Rapunzel, the fairytale princess whose prince climbed up her strong, beautiful hair to the tower where she was held prisoner to rescue her.

I think you will all agree that hair is a woman's crowning glory. It's mine. It's the crown we wear to show how we feel about ourselves.

Martin Luther so appropriately stated it: *The hair is the richest ornament of women.*

No matter the current fad, beautiful hair is always in fashion. When we know our hair is beautiful, it makes us feel younger, more alive and more sensual. Fabulous hair makes a statement. It tells others you're healthy and admire who you are.

Hair is a very personal thing. Witness how one feels when there's a "bad hair day" or when one has a bad haircut. "Bad hair" sets the mood for the day or in the case of a bad haircut–weeks or months until it grows out.

In the 1950's ratted, sprayed, plastered-looking hair was considered "fashionable." That was from a woman's point of view. Ask any man and they will tell you they prefer soft, flowing hair. Whether you're interested in capturing a man's heart or not, it's a fact, by survey, he prefers silky hair he can run his fingers through and admire, whether your hair is long or short.

The next thing discovered by surveying American men is that many of them say hair is one of the first physical features they notice. If a woman's hair is beautiful, they're captivated. If it's lackluster, it's a turn-off. A shiny, healthy head of hair, just like a sweet smile, stops a man in his tracks.

My husband first fell in love with me from the back when my hair was waist-length. He would never admit it was my long, gorgeous hair that enchanted him but I knew it was true.

What's more delightful than silky, luscious locks you're proud to have your man run his fingers through or looking at yourself in the mirror proud to say your hair is your Crowning Glory?

If you're having a bad-hair day, bad-hair week or bad-hair decade, there's hope. You don't have to be a fanatic like I am but it will require dedication, patience and persistence. Your hair will not grow nor get thicker in a day.

Give it time, be patient and apply what you learn here and it will be healthier, thicker and more beautiful. Then you'll have those luscious locks for the rest of your life as long as you apply what works. And you won't have to do constant damage-control.

My Personal Hair Nightmares

To begin with, I'm going to tell you two stories so you won't feel like you're the only one who's been through the nightmare of hair loss, thin or thinning hair. As you've already read, during my teens I had hair that wouldn't grow, hair that was thin and lifeless. Later I lost over half my head of hair.

Here's what I did and what I learned about hair-growth as a result of the experiences I'm about to tell you.

First, I made an uncompromising decision. I didn't know how I was going to get the head of hair I wanted but I knew I would never give up.

I decided to stop worrying about it. I knew if I worried, it wouldn't get me anywhere. I had to find out what I didn't know, apply what worked and discard the rest. There were other women around with the thick, gorgeous mane of hair I wanted, so I knew it was possible.

I started finding my answers in a most surprising way, a way I had no idea would result in getting the answers I needed.

Here is my first experience. Prepare yourself–it's different.

When I was nineteen I was hospitalized with a ruptured appendix. A year later I had a pain in my right ovary that wouldn't go away. When the pain was at its worst, I finally went to a doctor. He discovered I had a cyst in my right ovary the size of a grapefruit and told me I needed to get into surgery immediately or it could rupture.

Now here I am very clearly making a disclaimer. In no way am I recommending anyone do what I did. The purpose in my telling you this story is not for you to follow in my footsteps if you have a similar condition, but for you to read to the end of the story so you'll know what I personally learned about hair-growth.

When the doctor told me I needed surgery I thought to myself, "I'm not going to allow my body to be cut into again. Tomorrow someone is going to hand me the answer to this." At peace with myself, I walked out of his office with the doctor thinking I was crazy. Believe it or not, during the rest of that day, I forgot all about it.

Later the next day a friend walked up to me, showed me a book on natural healing and asked me if I'd read it. I said no and asked to borrow it. It was primarily a book on fasting. I knew nothing about natural remedies and didn't even know there was such a thing.

I turned to the index and looked up "cysts." It said that the formation of a cyst is a mechanism to protect the body from toxins and recommended the way to get rid of it was to fast on carrot juice. It explained that carrot juice is chemically the closest in makeup to our own blood and it contains every nutrient the body needs, except protein. So I decided to fast.

I fasted for nineteen days on water. I don't remember why I decided to fast on water first, but I did. (If a fast is undertaken it should be done under strict medical supervision.) I was very brave (and maybe stupid) in those days. Or maybe we can just chalk it up to naivety.

While I was fasting, the pain was increasing but different than what it was before. It was a strong pulling sensation. I lost weight and the cyst went down to about the size of a golf ball.

After the water fast, I spent four months with a friend who owned property in the San Ynez Mountains north of Santa Barbara, California.

Now for those Baby Boomers who were part of the hippy era, this won't come as a surprise. My friend and I lived off wild herbs and vegetables, a little brown rice and maybe an egg once a week. The main staple of the diet was a quart of fresh carrot juice daily. I decided to live this way for as long as it took until the cyst was gone.

Every day my body was drenched in clean, clear sunlight. I bathed and washed my hair in a beautiful little stream with a small waterfall. (My mother would be appalled if she knew all this. She raised me to be a complete lady, not a wild woman living in the hills eating watercress out of a river.)

Now keep in mind, I had no attention on my hair at all. During those four months I never combed my hair out even though it was always washed and clean. And I never looked in a mirror. One thing was for sure, four months earlier my hair was shoulder-length; it had refused to grow and was thin and wispy.

At the end of those four months, the pain was gone. I decided to go back to the doctor. Before my visit, I took a real shower at the Santa Barbara Harbor so I didn't look like a jungle woman when I walked into his office.

I took my shower. Then as I started combing the tangles out of my hair, something very strange and new was occurring. As the tangles were

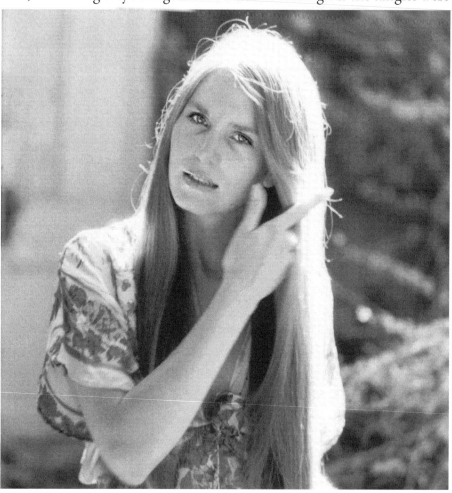

coming out one by one, my hair seemed to grow inches and then feet. Of course it wasn't growing at the time I was standing there. It already had. The length of my hair had gone from the top of my shoulders to my waist in four months.

I then took my first look in the mirror and hardly recognized the reflection. My eyes were as clear as blue sapphires. My skin was flawless with a soft, golden-brown glow. And my hair, my glorious hair was gleaming with shine and twice as thick as it had been four months earlier. It was a dazzling golden mane to my waist! I was finally Rapunzel. And stunned!

I then hurried to make my appointment with the doctor. The one I had seen four months earlier wasn't there so I saw another doctor in the practice. With a very confused expression on his face, he looked at the original records and without being able to look me in the eye, said, "I don't know what Dr. _____ was talking about. You never had a cyst in the first place." That was the only way he could possibly explain the "disappearance" of the cyst.

That moment was my wake-up call to natural healing. And the biggest unexpected bonus was the dream of long, lush hair becoming a reality. Carrot juice, sunshine, healthy food–who would have thought! I certainly had had no idea. But there it was, a gorgeous mane of to-live-for-hair. It was truly exhilarating!

A few years later...

My hip-length gorgeous hair remained the envy of every woman.

In truth, I was getting tired of my hair being that long. It kept getting caught in door jambs. But as my husband loved it so much, I kept it long for him.

To tell you just how much he loved it, one day he appeared at our front door looking pathetic and wouldn't even enter our own house. He said to me, with a big elephant tear running down his cheek, "You thought of cutting your hair today, didn't you?" He even knew I was thinking about cutting if off! What was a wife to do? Cut her hair and see her husband cry every day?

Fast forward to a few months later...part two of the saga...

I got very sick with pneumonia with a 104 degree temperature for several days. After I recuperated, my hair started falling out in massive handfuls due to the depletion my body went through. As you can well imagine, I was completely panicked. After all I went through to grow this incredible mane, now my hair was going to fall out like this!? I don't think so! I wanted my hair shorter, but to fall out like this? No way!

I frantically looked through the yellow pages for a scalp and hair specialist. I found one in the heart of West Hollywood and dashed there, hoping for a miracle; that somehow he could glue my hair back on or something. I didn't care. Something! My husband was going to be a sobbing, slobbering mess of tears!

Well! At a million words a minute I explained everything to Joe, my scalp specialist. He very calmly laid my head back into a sink to wash my hair. Remember, my hair is over three feet long and his sink is only a foot deep at the most. In other words, it was a challenge to wash all that hair in that small sink. Bear with me... we're almost at the crisis of the century. I'm just painting the picture...

So! Joe is done washing my hair. As I'm pulling my head up from the sink to sit upright in the chair, I notice that there seems to be a peculiar weight at the back of my neck. I put my hand back there to find out what was happening and went into shock! My entire head of hair, what was left of it, was in one enormous, humongous tangled knot. One big, fat knot!

Joe stared at this "knot" (which looked like a porcupine) with the blood in his face running to his feet, went to his phone and cancelled his appointments for the rest of the day. I knew someday I would be able to laugh about this whole scenario. But this certainly wasn't the day.

We sat looking at each other mirror-image; stunned and speechless. Poor guy, pale as a ghost, went to his refrigerator and pulled out two items: a giant-size bottle of safflower oil and a quart of mayonnaise. I'm looking at this and thinking, "Is there something I'm missing here, a bottle of safflower oil and a quart of mayonnaise! What? Are you kidding!"

Joe then proceeded to pour the entire bottle of safflower oil on the knot to try to disentangle it. After that didn't work, he took the mayonnaise and globbed it on by the handful. I was beginning to feel like a salad. After two to three hours of Joe and I just barely being able to get the ends out of the massive knot, I knew I needed to call my husband.

Now, I told you earlier how he felt about my long, beautiful hair. Needless to say, I wasn't looking forward to calling him and saying "Honey, your wife's hair is in a big, fat knot that isn't coming out. Please come help."

When he arrived he was wonderful and reassuring. Believe it or not, he worked with Joe for an additional seven hours attempting to get the stubborn knot out.

At 11:00 PM, we all looked at the scissors, agreed, and the knot, instead of coming out, came off. The longest we could cut my hair was shoulder-length. If it was cut any longer it would have looked like a freak hairdo with no plan to it as it was a million different lengths from being in an unmovable knot.

After it all got chopped off, I looked at my husband to see if his vision of me as his "Rapunzel" had burst but thank goodness, if it did, he didn't let it show. He was a real hero about it and still loved me.

Joe was panicked I would sue him for some silly reason. I knew the infamous knot was due to my hair having lost its elasticity because of my body's depletion, not because of something he did.

This is where the miracle happened–again. (Remember the first miracle of how my hair grew almost two feet in four months?)

I received scalp and hair treatments from Joe once a week for the next three months. Right from the beginning, hair started sprouting out of my head. (You know how fast grass grows after a rain? Like that.) At first I had a "butch" all over my head. It was pretty weird. Half my hair was shoulder-length and the other half was one inch in length, growing straight up!

During those next three months new hair grew in rapidly. Within six months, my hair was almost to my waist again.

Now, what was the magic Joe performed to set in motion amazing hair-growth and make it even healthier?

Two things:

1. His shampoo and conditioner had oil in them! I'm sure you're thinking, "How can oil clean the hair?" But it did. And my hair looked phenomenal and even thicker than before!

I kept pushing him to market his products but he'd say, "Jeanne, no one's going to want to buy these products because they have to be shaken up before use." No matter how many times I told him that was ridiculous, he wouldn't budge. I've tried to find Joe many times in the last 20 years, but to no avail.

So the question I've had to answer on my own was, "Which oils to use?"

Through personal research and years of experience I have discovered the specific beneficial oils to be used on the hair and those just for the scalp itself. This information is included in the following chapters. I know, without any doubt, the oils I will tell you about help make hair grow, look healthier, thicker and shinier.

2. Now the big one. Joe sprayed minerals on my scalp and massaged them in for 20-30 minutes, bringing nutrition to the follicles and oxygen and circulation to the scalp.

I'm sure you've experienced what it's like when you've been to a beautiful place and taken in deep breaths of crystal clear pure air. The oxygen rejuvenates not only your whole body, but *you* also.

The later section on scalp massage and slant boards gives the procedures on how to get oxygen flowing into your scalp and body. That, in addition to taking enough minerals (chapter on Diet) and using specific oils is key.

Oils, minerals and the flow of oxygen through massage! I was starting to understand even more of the basic elements of hair growth.

I hope the story I just told was informative and entertaining. In looking back, I was able to laugh to myself about what happened, *especially* since my hair became even thicker and stronger after that.

One day, after you've read and applied the information contained in this book, you will look back and be happy, too.

Let's take that thinning or thin, lifeless hair that refuses to grow and turn it into a crown you're proud to wear!

Are you ready to let your light shine, inside and out?

I hope you've answered with a resounding, "Yes!"

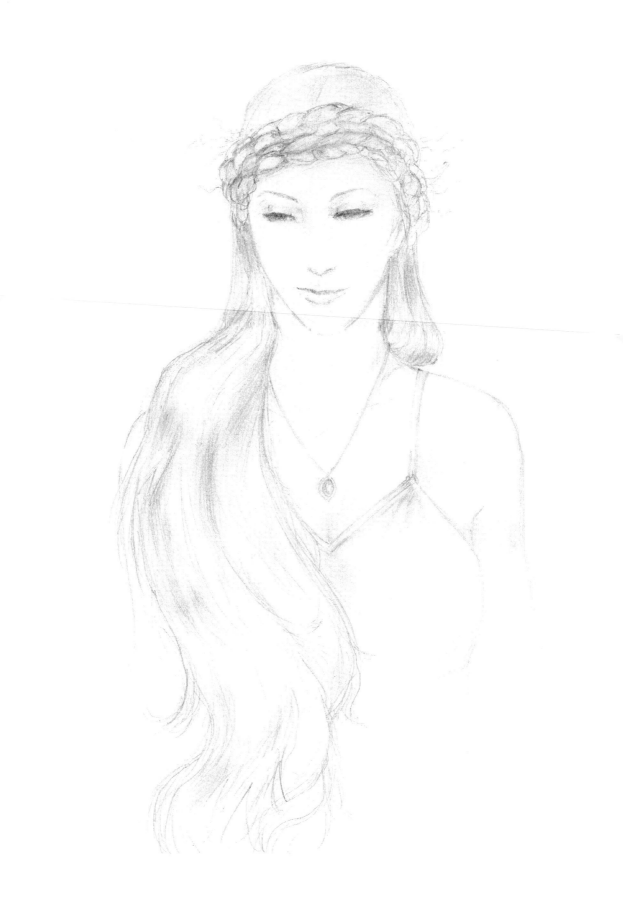

Chapter Two

What to Do to Have Beautiful Hair!

"Would that they had been curls, the twist of sunlight caught in their luxurious depth may have been blinding, a circumstance that the angels themselves no doubt forbade."

Bart Gangemi

Up until the mid-nineteenth century women mostly wore their hair long. Their hair was thick and beautiful and remained that way. How did they manage to have such gorgeous hair? It was simple; pure, whole nutrition along with few, if any, toxins in their environment and food.

My purpose here is to give you simple techniques that make sense rather than "one-shot, quick-fix" solutions in a bottle full of chemical ingredients. The quick-fix mentality is exactly what has driven the chemical culture that created the problems in the first place.

Some of the chemically-based products in broad use today are creating alarming side-effects.

A highly respected nutritionist told me about a toxic ingredient used as a preservative in most hair and skin products, an ingredient found to be dangerous to a regulatory gland in the body. Absorption of this toxic ingredient can lead to depression and a myriad of other appalling symptoms. I'll be talking more about that and other ingredients later.

The scalp, just like the rest of the skin on the body, absorbs what is applied to it. That includes shampoos, conditioners, hairsprays, gels and chemical hair-growth products.

Research has discovered that toxic chemicals absorbed into the body through the skin can create problems in overall health over the long term. One then has to "solve" those problems, just as one may have tried to solve a hair problem with a chemical product, causing more damage and problems with the hair later on.

It's an endless cycle of damage-control.

These quick-fix solutions, as in chemical hair-growth products, sometimes give instant gratification and results. Unfortunately the use of chemical products can, over time, result in damage, loss of hair and premature aging. Strong statement, I know.

Again...all that has changed since the era where women had beautiful hair without effort is due to a) the toxins we consume, b) the toxic chemicals we put on our hair, scalp and skin, and c) the quality of food and nutrition.

We now have to reverse the trend and get back to what works. It's not complicated. But it can take a while to undo the damage and restore the natural balance.

Why replace long-term overall health and well-being with toxic solutions? If we desire to live a long life, look and feel great, we must listen to Mother Nature.

Women spend an average of $1,500 a year on hair-care and hair products which don't get the needed long-term results. Most people think the more money spent on a product, the more superior it is. That's not always true unless it comes from unique hard-to-find natural sources or a specific proprietary formulation.

Know that just because it's inexpensive doesn't mean it's ineffective. I'm going to show you how to look good *and* save a lot of money!

Here are the three proven steps for an extremely effective and quick method to reverse the damage caused to your hair by toxic chemicals. If you can't get your hair to stay shiny, full and healthy-looking, this is what you can do for overnight help. Anyone who applies the following three steps will experience an astounding difference in their hair.

The Magic Overnight Hair Beautification Procedure!

STEP 1:

Get a chlorine shower filter! This is *essential* if you want your hair to be healthy (not to mention your whole body).

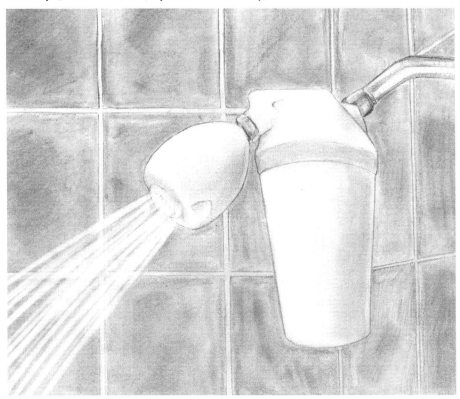

Anywhere one lives, especially a place with very toxic water, one is shocked to discover how clogged the filter is after six months of use. In Florida, where I've lived for several years, the water is filled with heavy metals, chlorine and many other toxic chemicals. With an effective filter the toxins are captured within the filter and not allowed to come into contact with the scalp and body.

Toxic build-up makes the hair look and feel like straw. With a good filter, there's little to no build-up to damage your hair, clog your scalp or get absorbed into your body. You will see and feel an amazing difference in the texture, shine and fullness of your hair and the softness of your skin after using a good chlorine filter.

Chlorine shower filters are available in department or hardware stores or can be ordered online. The cost varies. Not all chlorine shower filters are of the same quality. By far the best ones are those that have the actual filter lower than the shower head with a built-in water flow regulator. If the water pressure is too high while flowing through a filter, the filter cannot eliminate as many toxins as a filter that has a built-in water flow regulator.

Don't believe anyone who tells you that shower filters automatically eliminate 95% or more of the toxins. The only way a filter can be effective is if the following two things are done:

1) Keep the water pressure to a minimum while washing and rinsing your hair. (You don't have to be concerned about that if your shower filter has a built-in water-flow regulator) and,

2) keep the water temperature slightly warm or even a little bit cool. If there's too much water flowing through the filter at too high of a temperature, the filter cannot do the job it's intended to do.

The biggest additional benefit of keeping the water pressure and temperature low is that the outside layers of your hairs aren't getting stripped by heat and pressure.

You'll see a *major* difference in your hair when you follow those two guidelines.

See the "Products" section at www.themodernrapunzel.com for an excellent chlorine shower filter with the filter lower than the shower head and a built-in water regulator.

Now is a good time to give you one of the basics of hair structure to help you understand how chemicals affect the hair.

The outside layer, the part we see, is called the cuticle. The cuticle acts as a protective barrier for the inner structure of the hair.

Toxic chemicals and too much heat applied to the hair (blow drying, curling irons, flat irons and the sun) damage the cuticle, causing hair to be porous. Porous means something that has holes in it, something that allows infiltration of substances. When the hair is porous, toxic chemicals can penetrate the inside layers, harming them. Simply put, the more porous the hair, the more it soaks up toxins and the dryer and more damaged the hair becomes.

This makes the hair dull, rough and tangle easily due to cuticle damage. The more damaged the cuticle, the more the hair loses its "elasticity" making the hair vulnerable to breakage and hair-loss.

The word "elastic" means something that can return to its original state after being stretched. Over time, toxic water, chemical hair-care products and heat cause the hairs to lose their ability to bounce back.

The health of one's hair is determined by its elasticity.

Here's the test to determine how strong or weak a hair strand is:

THE ELASTICITY TEST

Pull a hair out of your head and using both hands, hold the hair at each end with the index finger and thumb. Pull the ends and then let it bounce back. How elastic is it? Does it stay stretched without bouncing back? Does it break?

If it's slow to bounce back, doesn't bounce back at all, breaks or stretches to double or more its original length, your hair is in trouble. Do not perm or color your hair until it has its elasticity restored. Otherwise you'll have a real mess later on that will be next to impossible to turn around.

If it bounces back and doesn't break, it's healthy.

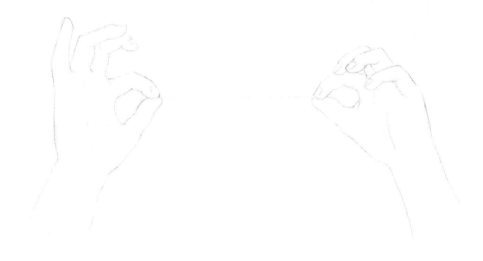

Do the elasticity test periodically to determine when it's safe to chemically process your hair.

When my hair was both permed and colored and before I started using a chlorine shower filter, it was gummy, horribly dry and at one point I had to cut it all off which was most upsetting! My hair had lost its elasticity from the toxic chemicals in the water and from being permed and colored all at the same time. When I started using a chlorine shower filter and applied the next two steps, it regained its elasticity and became shiny and luxurious.

I hope this test illustrates why it's so important to not only use a chlorine shower filter but to refrain from applying toxic hair-care products to the hair itself and protect your hair from too much heat. Later I will describe the kind of hair-care products to use and the procedures to apply to protect your hair from damage over the short and long-term.

Now that you're preventing future chemical build-up through the use of a filter, here's how you can remove any accumulated toxic build-up that has affected the elasticity and health of your hair:

STEP 2:

Get a gentle, non-toxic clarifying shampoo. "Clarify" in this sense means removing the majority or all of the accumulated toxic build-up on your hair through the use of a clarifying shampoo.

If you don't use chemical hair products and live in a rural area where the water is not as toxic, you won't need to use a clarifier as often. But if your hair is not shiny and thicker after doing Steps 1 and 3 (Step 3 coming up), then periodically use a clarifier.

When your hair starts to feel even a little heavy and is losing its shine, you'll know it's time. On the average, I use a clarifier once or twice a month depending on the environment I'm in and how my hair feels.

After using a good clarifier, you'll notice that your hair has a lot more bounce and the color is much more alive.

Some of the clarifiers on the market are very harsh and strip not only the toxins out of the hair, but the natural oils as well. Make sure you get a gentle, natural clarifying shampoo. Even then it's best to first combine the clarifier with a regular chemical-free shampoo on your palms before applying, especially if your hair is fragile.

Clarifying your hair will make an *enormous* difference!

See the "Products" section at www.themodernrapunzel.com for gentle and natural clarifying shampoos, regular shampoos and conditioners.

Just before the "Charts" section in the back of the book are two step-by-step procedures on a) how to use a clarifying shampoo when there's heavy chemical build-up and b) how to make and apply your own home-made clarifier when there's no heavy chemical build-up. This method removes the residual shampoo that if left in the hair can make the hair dry.

STEP 3:

Here's what to do to restore the elasticity of your hair now that it's free of toxic build-up. It is accomplished by applying certain oils to your hair.

This step is implemented when your hair is completely dry.

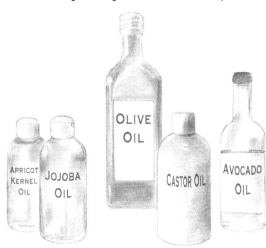

As a quick note first: jojoba and castor oil are used on the scalp to help with thinning hair. Later I will be going over why these specific oils are applied to the scalp and the procedure for applying them.

For our purposes now of restoring the elasticity, strength and health of the hair, I'm giving you the list of oils to apply to *only the hair itself.*

The oils to be applied to the hair and not the scalp *at this time* are:
Apricot kernel oil,
Jojoba oil,
Coconut oil,
Avocado oil,
Extra virgin olive oil.

These are listed in order of lightest to heaviest in terms of how much conditioning your hair needs. You can obtain these organic, cold-pressed oils at your local health-food store.

I've had several women ask about combining the oils. I like applying each one individually so I know which oil is getting the results I want. Do your own experimenting. Everyone's hair is a little different according to its degree of dryness and how fine or coarse it is.

Make sure the oils are cold-pressed, organic and haven't been sitting on the shelf for a long time. Just like any oil, they can go rancid. To test for rancidity, place a little of the oil on the back of your tongue. If it burns, it's rancid. The oil will also smell a little sharp or "off" if it's rancid.

APRICOT KERNEL OIL

Apricot kernel oil is used by the Hunza people in India on their skin and hair. They also take it internally. The women, at the age of 80, barely have a wrinkle on their faces and have beautiful, shiny, healthy hair.

JOJOBA OIL

Here's what a Cosmetologist has to say about jojoba oil:

> *"Jojoba oil is very close in molecular structure to the natural oil of the scalp. That's why it's such a good conditioner for the hair and scalp. The molecules are tiny so they can actually penetrate the hair shaft. As we age, we have less and less natural oil that is produced by the scalp, so our hair will frequently get drier, especially after menopause. This is mainly due to a lack of circulation to the scalp. One of the special qualities about jojoba oil is that it is not really "oil" at all but is more like a liquid wax. Sebum, a liquid wax, found naturally in human skin (especially on the scalp), acts to waterproof and protect both hair and skin, keeping skin from becoming dry and brittle. It also can control the growth of microorganisms on the skin. Because jojoba is so similar to sebum, it easily mimics the same functions."*

Jojoba oil is the best oil for crisis handling. It absorbs completely into the hair shaft which makes each individual hair softer and thicker.

COCONUT OIL

Coconut oil is known for its rich healing properties. It has many uses, one of which is a wonderful emollient (softening and soothing) for the hair.

AVOCADO AND EXTRA VIRGIN OLIVE OILS

If my hair is especially dry, I use avocado or extra virgin olive oil. Both are fabulous for restoring condition to damaged, over-processed hair.

Everyone's hair is different and will respond differently to different oils at different times. That's why it's good to keep all of them on hand. If one doesn't do the deep conditioning needed, another will.

Jojoba and apricot kernel oils are not so thick that they can't be washed out fairly easily. Coconut, avocado and olive oils are more difficult to wash out but so worth it in terms of shine and hair strength. You will see.

I suggest starting with jojoba oil. Apply lightly to the hair, not the scalp. There's no need to saturate your hair with it. Just make sure you have the oil throughout your hair, especially the driest parts, which are usually the crown, sides and ends. Let the oil absorb into your hair for half an hour to an hour (no longer) before you wash it.

I like sitting in the sauna with my hair uncovered. I put my hair up in a clip to keep it out of my face. One of those old-fashioned hair dryers with a hood works, too. With the oil in your hair, put the setting on low and leave your head under the hood for about a half an hour, no more. Make sure the heat is comfortably warm, definitely not hot, especially on the scalp. The heat from a sauna or this kind of a hair dryer allows the oil to penetrate even more. Remember to apply the oil to the hair only, not the scalp at this time.

When you apply one of these oil procedures to your hair, a) sitting in a sauna or b) using an old-fashioned hair dryer, you'll know how dry your hair was previously by how much oil has absorbed into your hair. If there's still a thick residue of oil left on your hair, you either put on too much or your hair wasn't exceptionally dry. Adjust the amount of oil you use according to how much it has absorbed into your hair. You may need to use a little more or a little less.

Wash your hair afterwards but do *not* shampoo all the oil out to the point where your hair is squeaky clean. *Never*, no matter what, wash your hair so that it feels squeaky clean. You don't want to make the hair dry out again or defeat the purpose of the oil. You can leave a very light residue of the oil in your hair for a couple of days which will continue the conditioning. The rest will come out in the next couple of washings.

You'll still need to apply a small amount of a moisturizing conditioner after shampooing out most of the oil, especially if your hair is long and has tangles that don't come out smoothly and easily. The extra conditioning will allow your comb to glide through your hair, which is what you want.

As you continue to apply this procedure, each individual hair will get stronger and thicker. This procedure will also help handle "fly-a-way" and frizzy hair. By doing this, you'll notice that you won't have to use heavy conditioners anymore.

If your hair is extremely damaged, apply one of the oils for a half hour to an hour before washing your hair about once a week. If your hair is not damaged, once every two weeks is good for maintenance. The degree of dryness will tell you how often you need to apply the oil. Applying the oils more often than what I've mentioned is not necessary and may cause your hair to become too gummy.

Remember, dry and processed hair is porous, meaning that it literally has holes in the hairs. Now that the chemicals have been removed from the cuticle by implementing the first two steps, the oils will give your hair the real strengthening it needs. You'll see that each individual hair will get thicker from this process. The oils plump up each hair so it looks and feels like you have more hair overall.

To fully get that elasticity back, use your favorites of these oils for as long as you need to. It's good to alternate them.

Do the elasticity test from time to time to determine when it's safe to process your hair with color or a perm.

These steps, done in sequence, do more for the hair as an instant and long-term handling for dryness and for damage than anything I've ever seen or experienced personally. Try it exactly as written and see for yourself. Even if your hair is in great shape, it's a good idea to follow this procedure to keep it that way.

Let me recap the steps of the Magic Overnight Hair Beautification Procedure:

1. Get, install and use a chlorine filter,
2. Clarify your hair with a gentle chemical-free clarifying shampoo,
3. Apply organic oil(s) obtained from your health food store.

SHINE!

The procedure you just read will help give your hair much more shine!

Another great technique to give shine to the hair after it's dry is to place a very small amount (a sixteenth to an eighth of a teaspoon, less or more, depending on how long your hair is) of either apricot kernel or coconut oil on your hands and then lightly smooth your hair with your hands. It will calm down the frizzies and give a great feel. Make sure you use a very small amount.

Again, remember that having a chlorine filter using medium-low water pressure and slightly warm, never hot, water will also make a tremendous difference in the shine and health of your hair.

Okay, let's now look at the reasons for hair loss and what to do about it.

Chapter Three

Chief Causes of Hair Loss

According to the American Academy of Dermatology, at least two-thirds of American women struggle with thinning hair.

From my own experience and research, I have discovered that the first eight causes listed below are the top offenders of hair loss. Each one is covered extensively in this book.

The last four pertain to individual situations and there may be other rare and isolated ones. If that's the case you will need to see a competent health-care practitioner.

No matter what, you will acquire vast benefits by reading, understanding and applying the basics in this book to help regain your head of hair.

Here are the primary reasons for hair loss and thinning hair:

- Stress
- Lack of proper circulation to the scalp resulting in clogged follicles*
- Use of chemical products on the scalp resulting in clogged follicles
- Hair that has lost its elasticity† due to toxic chemicals and heat

---

* follicle: a very small hole in the skin from where hair grows. The hairs grow within the follicles until they exit the scalp. The scalp contains hundreds of hair follicles every square inch.

† elasticity: the ability of a hair to stretch easily and then return to its original shape quickly.

- ❧ Lack of proper nutrition
- ❧ Hormonal problems
- ❧ Toxins
- ❧ Illness which has depleted the stores of nutrients in the body
- ❧ Under or over-active thyroid in which case you need to be tested by a competent health-care practitioner
- ❧ Some medicines
- ❧ Certain infections
- ❧ Chemotherapy

Before addressing unnatural hair loss, let's take a look at:

"Natural Hair Loss"

There is a lot of controversy on how many hairs fall out naturally. Some experts say a normal amount is 50-100 hairs a day. I feel that's a guess. Most of the year I lose on the average 15-20 hairs a day as a result of applying the procedures contained in this book.

Keep in mind, the human body follows the same pattern (hair loss) as animals (fur loss) in the summer. At some point, in spring or summer, animals start to shed their winter coats. It's the same with most human bodies, except our bodies shed hair.

For a month or two each spring or summer, I can lose up to 50 hairs a day. And then it returns to the normal amount of 15-20 hairs a day.

There's no need to panic when you notice an unusual amount of hair coming out once a year. The important thing is to ensure that your scalp is replacing those hairs that have fallen out.

Keep reading...

Chapter Four

How to Prevent and Stop Hair Loss Naturally!

his section is extensive. Within this chapter are many important details to know, understand and apply. My objective is
to provide you with everything I've personally discovered
and researched in growing a full head of hair. By referring back to this
comprehensive section as often as needed, you will be availing yourself of
the complete picture and understanding in order to apply the techniques
successfully.

1. THE MAGIC OVERNIGHT HAIR BEAUTIFICATION PROCEDURE (SEE CHAPTER 2)

This begins the process of healthy hair and helps maintain it for a lifetime.

2. GET RID OF SPLIT ENDS

When the end of the hair starts to split, it continues to do so until the
hair is so compromised it breaks off. Liken it to a rope. If you've ever seen
the end of a rope that is frayed, you will see it keeps fraying; the rope gets
thinner and thinner until it eventually breaks.

That's what occurs when hair is split, but just because the end is split doesn't mean the rest of the hair is unhealthy, just the part that is split! By getting rid of split ends, those hairs have a chance; they will not fray and break off.

I have known women with long hair who won't cut their split ends. As a result their hair gets thinner and thinner as the years go by.

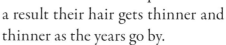

Many years ago I talked a friend of mine into cutting six inches of split and dry ends off her waist-length thinning hair. I promised her she would not only lose less hair but she would also start to grow more hair from her scalp and her hair would grow much faster. Although it was not without concern, she took the leap of faith.

Within a year after those ends were cut off, her hair was the thickness of what she had wanted for a long time. It had grown again to her waist but this time it looked completely different. It went from scraggly to a thick, gorgeous mane of hair all the way to her waist!

Have you ever noticed how alive your hair feels after a haircut with all those split ends gone? For me, it feels like my hair is thanking me.

When there are no split ends you'll be amazed at how much thicker your hair will get and how it will remain that way. And once it's long, it will be long and thick, not long and thin. What a wonderful simple thing to do! It requires patience until your hair gets to the length you want, but then all good things require patience.

So, if you have split ends, cut them off. *All of them!* Regardless of whether you have your hairstyle short or long, those ends need to come off now.

Let me share a great trick with you. If the ends of your hair are dry and not split, here's what you can do so they don't eventually split. Take equal amounts of jojoba oil and pure vitamin E oil or castor oil, combine on your palms and then saturate the dry ends with this mixture. It will be very sticky and thick. Leave the mixture on those ends for an hour or two, then shampoo, condition and voilà, little to no dry ends! As a result of doing this, not only are you saving those ends from splitting and eventually having to be cut off, you're naturally reversing the damage.

3. BRUSHING AND MASSAGE

The scalp needs some help!

Once a person's head has been balding for some time it can become difficult to revive the follicles and reverse the process, but it can be done with determination.

This section is *key* in helping revive the follicles. Lack of circulation to the scalp is a major cause of hair loss and inhibition of new hair growth.

Circulation to the scalp is accomplished through brushing and scalp massage which stimulate the flow of blood. As a result, nutrition from the blood can now feed the hair follicles.

BRUSHING

Generally speaking, the top of the head is the most important part of a woman's hairstyle. Most women brush and comb their scalp as part of their daily routine. By doing this, the nerves and muscles attached to the scalp glands are being worked, thus making them function normally. If the nerves, muscles and scalp glands are not worked or massaged, thinning or baldness can occur.

If your hair is thin on top despite brushing, don't lose hope. Coming up are other methods to grow in new hair.

THE SAFE WAY TO BRUSH YOUR HAIR

Brush your hair only when it's dry. Never, ever brush it when it's wet or damp in the slightest. It's ideal to use a boar bristle brush. No matter what kind of brush you use make sure the tips don't snag your hair. They have to be perfectly smooth. Stay away from brushes that have a double bristle— one long and one short—as those kinds of brushes can tear the hair.

After your hair is completely dry and any tangles are gently combed out, lightly brush your hair upside-down starting from the back of the neck and continue brushing to the top of the head, all the while remaining upside-down. Always ensure you don't yank the hair as it may be a little tangled from being upside-down. Continue brushing until you feel the circulation throughout your scalp. This usually takes less than a minute. Then right-side-up, brush it gently again starting from the bottom.

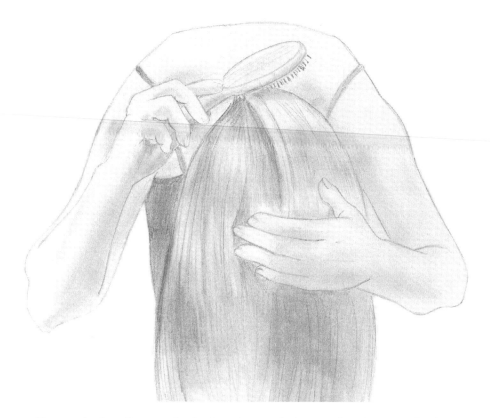

Be gentle, but firm with the brushing while your head is upside-down. You don't need to brush a lot, just enough daily brushing to keep the circulation going. You will know. Too much brushing can make the scalp overly sensitive, so be aware of that.

If you're finding a lot of hair in your brush after brushing it, there's always the temptation of being careful in doing *anything* with your hair. Know you're getting much needed circulation to the follicles when you brush and massage your scalp for a short time daily. The scalp needs loving communication, not fear. While you're brushing or massaging, lightly and with love, tell your scalp to grow hair. It works.

If your hair is curly, brushing can make it too bushy. In that case, the way to get circulation to the scalp is through massage while using a slant board, which is discussed later.

MASSAGE

I'm sure we can agree that massage makes us feel great. The benefits of massage are vast.

Let me provide you with a short description of what a "follicle" is and what scalp massage has to do with it.

A follicle is a small hole in the scalp from which the hair grows. Hairs grow within the follicles until they exit the scalp. The scalp contains hundreds of follicles every square inch.

Massage, whether manually or with an electric massager, accomplishes two things in helping hair break through the follicle: 1) it helps dislodge any hairs that have become trapped in the follicle and 2) helps dislodge debris from the empty hair follicles. As a result of the increased circulation and blood supply, new hair is spun and the hairs are now able to break through the follicles as they are not clogged with debris.

An electrical massager is great for these purposes.

See the "Products" section at www.themodernrapunzel.com for where to obtain an electric massager and a small hand-held manual massager.

The three ways we've gone over so far in getting circulation to your scalp are:
1. Brushing
2. Hand massage (The section on slant boards will give you the detailed massage procedure for opening the follicles to grow in new hair.)
3. Massage with an electric massager

Here's the fourth and final way:

The scalp should freely move over the skull. If it doesn't, circulation is impeded and the follicles aren't getting vital oxygen and blood. Follicles must have oxygen and blood to grow new hair.

To test how tight your scalp is, grab some hair right next to the scalp, hold it firmly and then gently pull that bunch of hair up and down. Can you feel your scalp move freely and easily across the skull? If not, here's what you can do:

   a. Spread your fingers and run them into a section of your hair next to the scalp

   b. Grab the hair in that section

   c. While holding your hair securely, gently pull the hair up, down and then sideways for a few seconds until you feel your scalp move

   d. Do this on your whole head for a few seconds on each area

   e. Depending on how tight your scalp is, you can do this procedure one or more times a day for a total of a minute each time

This is an additional technique which helps increase circulation to the scalp

MORE UNDERSTANDING

Attached to the follicles are oil glands. These oil glands lubricate the inside walls of the follicles. If the oil glands secrete too much oil, the follicles can become clogged.

Sweat glands are next to the follicles. If the sweat glands work as they should, the scalp is fine. If they over-produce, the salt in our own perspiration strips the hair of its natural oils, resulting in dry, flyaway hair. Excess perspiration can also bring pollutants into the follicles and add to the blockage if the scalp is not properly cleaned, brushed and massaged.

There are also nerves and muscles in every square inch of the scalp. These nerves and muscles are attached to the oil and sweat glands.

Massage, whether manually or with an electrical massager, stimulates the nerves and muscles attached to the sweat and oil glands which make the glands produce normal, not excessive, quantities of oil and perspiration. *Normalizing the quantities of oil and perspiration is very important for hair growth.*

Brushing and massage will also help decrease or eliminate an excessively oily scalp.

I recommend daily brushing and the gentle use of an electric massager one to two times a week for less than a minute each time. This helps ensure the oil and sweat glands are functioning properly.

4. FREE UP CONGESTION IN THE FOLLICLES

Here is the information on what oils to apply to your scalp and why:

Dr. Ian Shillington, a noted Naturopathic Doctor, told me of the great benefits of castor oil. For six months, one of his previously bald-headed patients nightly massaged certified organic castor oil into his scalp. That, along with a nutrient-dense product called "Total Nutrition," restored a full head of hair to his male patient. I will talk more about that later.

Castor oil breaks up congestion in any part of the body, which includes the hair follicles. Jojoba oil will also break up congestion although not quite as effectively as castor oil. The advantage of jojoba oil is that it's easier to wash out.

The most effective and detailed method of scalp massage for thin, thinning or balding hair, with or without oils, is coming up in the chapter "Slant Boards: The Most Vital Piece of Equipment You'll Ever Own."

TOO MUCH OIL CAN CLOG THE FOLLICLES

Many Italians use olive oil on their scalps, east Indians use coconut oil, Africans use palm oil. People from these countries have naturally over-producing oil glands. Adding more oil to the scalp causes more hair loss as the follicles are getting more and more clogged. Those who consume a diet of cooked oils and fatty animal products could also have more of a tendency toward hair loss.

For those with oily hair, in addition to the hundreds of oil glands that exist on every square inch on the scalp, oil applied to the scalp can be too much. Excess oil can attract debris into the follicles, clogging them and preventing new hair from reaching the surface.

Also, if your scalp is oily try cutting out fried foods completely and use a massager on your scalp.

For those with oily hair it's *always* safe to brush and massage without oil and apply the other procedures in this book.

Through a regimen of:

- daily light brushing and combing,
- once or twice weekly use of a massager on the scalp for one minute, and,

❧ applying the scalp-massage procedure on a slant board, with or without oil,

...new hairs will be encouraged to grow and break through.

5. LIMIT CHEMICAL PROCESSING AND AVOID USING CHEMICAL HAIR PRODUCTS

HAIR COLOR

If you're going to perm your hair do not color it also, or give it at the least one to two months between the two processes.

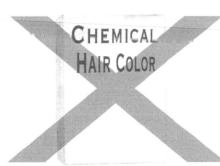

Do the elasticity test first before you perm or color your hair. *Remember, coloring and perming affect the elasticity of the hair big-time!*

Use the oils as described to restore elasticity. Your hair must be in fantastic shape before it's processed.

When you're ready for the roots to be colored, just color the roots, not the rest of the hair. Repeated coloring over the same hair is a sure way to cause permanent damage. At that point the only thing one can do is cut it all off. Re-growing one's whole head of hair takes time, is major aggravation and can be a blow to the pride of one's appearance.

Have your hairdresser keep an exact record of the brand-name and color of the product so the same color can be used on the roots each time.

It is my understanding that the only hair color that is truly organic is red henna. All others have chemical dyes added to them. Try to find a salon that uses hair color with as few chemicals as possible. Always check out the product ingredients. It's your hair and your health. Be ruthless.

If you color your own hair, hair-coloring products are available at most health-food stores. They're great and are also effective in covering gray.

Spend time studying the color charts on the back of the box so you know which one will work for your hair. To be safe, I suggest doing a strand test first. Write down the brand name and the color once you've found the right one.

PERMANENTS

If your hair is falling out, do not perm your hair no matter how tempting it is. I know that perms are done to compensate for thin hair in the desire to have the appearance of full hair, but it's a huge mistake no matter what anyone tells you.

If hair is falling out, the health and elasticity has already been compromised. Why make it worse just for short-term fullness and curls?

Even if your hair is not thin, have you ever noticed your hair falls out more than usual after a perm? When the perm grows out, your hair will look thinner, because it is.

Get someone to give you a really good haircut to suit your face while you're implementing the other procedures. In the long run you'll be very, very happy you did.

WHEN YOUR HAIR IS IN SHAPE TO BE PERMED OR STRAIGHTENED

Once your hair has its elasticity and strength fully restored, you can perm your hair again. Again, please don't perm and color your hair at the same time.

Here are some suggestions from a cosmetologist on preventing the hair and scalp from being burned during perming:

> *"Have a timer on hand or bring one with you to the salon and always set the timer to avoid over-processing your hair and burning your scalp. Using a timer is safer than forgetting or relying on a busy hairdresser to check her watch."*

There really is no gentle perm. Unfortunately, a perm is a perm is a perm. The chemical, ammonium thioglycolate, is the only ingredient known thus far to actually alter the protein in the hair to change its structure from straight to curly or vice-versa.

Cosmetologists do not recommend perms done at home. The chemicals are way too strong and it's hard to predict what could happen. Only a competent hair-dresser knows how to handle the various situations that can come up.

PRODUCTS USED ON THE SCALP AND HAIR

Why is it important to use all-natural products instead of toxic chemically-based ones?

First, let's take a look at something vital to understand.

Many people self-diagnose and use products in a frantic effort to stop hair loss. Without enough knowledge of what certain products do, one can make oneself vulnerable to side-effects and eventual major health problems. Many of these medications and products contain toxic ingredients which can affect hormones and one's overall health.

Balanced hormones give emotional balance. Therefore, hormones out of balance create havoc emotionally and physically. Do you really want to have your hormones interfered with and deal with the consequences caused by toxic substances?

Fortunately, there are natural and very effective ways to help prevent hair loss and grow one's hair back. Yes, it takes longer, but the benefits are vast. When one goes the natural route, in addition to creating a healthy head of hair, one's overall health is also restored and maintained.

One has to look at the long-term benefits of the natural route versus the short-term toxic chemical route. The short-term route gives one a temporary sense of comfort and freedom from anxiety, but in the long-term it's disastrous. It's never fun to look back and say to yourself, "I should never have done that."

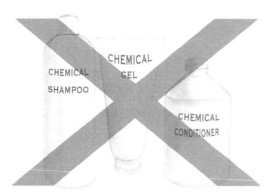

So where do we go from here? By combining massage and not allowing chemical products of any kind to touch your scalp, you have a very good chance at decreasing hair loss and increasing hair growth, if not eliminating hair loss completely in some cases.

IF YOU NEED TO USE HAIR SPRAYS

Use a pump spray, never aerosol and never spray hairspray or any kind of spray products directly onto your scalp, natural or not. When spraying, keep the spray pump far enough away from your scalp so the spray reaches your hair, not the scalp.

To style the hair on top of your head, hold or brush your hair up and spray the hair (not the roots) to hold the hair on top in place. You can also spray the hair spray onto your hand or brush, apply to your hair and comb or brush through. For a firm hold repeat several times. When spraying the sides of the head, cover the temple area with your other hand.

It may take some time to master this procedure but by following it you are protecting your scalp from damage and the follicles from getting clogged.

A good substitute for hair spray is a chemical-free gel which eliminates the possibility of hair spray coming into contact with your scalp.

Remember, chemicals damage the scalp and the outside layer of the hair, called the shaft. Find a chemical-free hair spray. Ensure that all your hair-care products are natural. Even when the products are natural, do not allow them to come into contact with your scalp, except shampoo.

MORE ON CLOGGED FOLLICLES

We've heard or read that follicles can die. But how is that possible if it's just a hole? If you get the idea of a follicle as a hole in the ground, it can get clogged with dirt and debris.

Every day we lose hairs from the follicles just by brushing, combing or natural fallout so that new hairs can take its place. Because that empty follicle is left open, clogging agents can seep in with your own excess oil or perspiration acting as a carrying agent, trapping the debris in the follicle.

The empty follicles don't become clogged all at one time. They collect debris in various amounts over time until the follicles are completely blocked. Then the hair growing beneath the debris is prevented from breaking through the scalp.

The use of oil-based shampoos and conditioners on the scalp can clog the pores except for natural oil-based shampoos specifically designed for thinning hair. There *are* some essential oils mixed in with hair-care products that are very effective at helping re-grow hair. You can find those shampoos and conditioners on my website.

To reiterate: Experts have said that overproducing oil or perspiration glands can be an important contributing cause of hair loss or baldness. Debris and chemical products (especially sticky ones) mix with the excess oil or perspiration produced in the scalp and may penetrate the hair follicles, clogging them.

Incorrect use of styling products and ineffective scalp cleaning are a major contributing factor to thinning hair. Spraying or rubbing sticky products on the hair and scalp has the same clogging effect on hair follicles that heavy makeup and creams have on facial pores and the entire body. The skin can't breathe which inhibits circulation. If a follicle is clogged, the hair can't make its way to the surface.

The ingredients in shampoos, conditioners, hair sprays and any other hair product can play a *big* part in the problem of hair loss whether used at home or in a salon.

Think back to the products you and your family have rubbed into your scalp since childhood. There may have been some unusual ones. Do you think it's possible a percentage of those products might still be trapped beneath the surface and stuck in the follicles? Know that they can be.

Deep-cleaning of the scalp removes trapped debris in the hair follicles. Along with castor and jojoba oils, there are some natural follicle detoxification products available. Ensure you follow the instructions.

See the "Products" section at www.themodernrapunzel.com for more follicle detoxification products besides jojoba and castor oils.

HOW TO SHAMPOO CORRECTLY

To shampoo, pour the shampoo onto the palm of one of your hands, work up a lather in both hands and then apply. Never pour the shampoo directly onto your scalp.

When visiting your hairdresser, don't let her massage your scalp with shampoo, as shampoo in contact with the scalp for more than a few seconds can disrupt the natural beneficial oils in the follicles. Ask her to massage with water only.

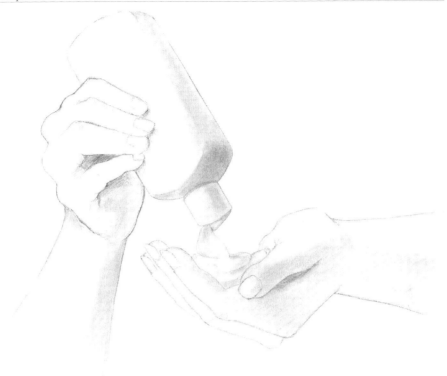

USE OF CONDITIONERS

Conditioners should only be placed on the hair, never on the scalp as they can clog the follicles.

6. ELIMINATE HAIR RESTRAINTS

Hair loss can occur from using ponytail holders, barrettes, pins or anything that restrains or binds hair for any length of time. Try not to use any of these hair items when you don't have to. In the case of ponytail holders, use cloth ones as they're not as tight.

Switch where you part your hair if you can. Maybe you've noticed that the place where you consistently part your hair is thinner than the other side. Change the part to another position now and then. It will help a lot.

WIGS

Scientists have often stated that an insufficient supply of blood flowing to the scalp may be the reason for hair loss. While thinning hair is somewhat easy to conceal by the use of wigs, wigs prevent the vital flow of blood and oxygen to the scalp. As a result, hair follicles cannot breathe, which prevents new hair from coming in.

HAIR WEAVING

The problem with hair weaving is the same as wigs; circulation. A wig can be removed and the scalp cleansed and rubbed each night, but not so with hair that is woven into your own hair. For that reason, hair weaving can be more damaging than wigs.

HAIR EXTENSIONS

Many people are reporting that hair extensions are not all they've been made out to be. It's possible to lose some natural hair from the scalp due to the extra weight of the extensions. Incorrect application or care of extensions can cause itching, pulling and breakage. Some people can experience allergies to the bonding glue.

The longer hair extensions are worn, the greater the danger can be. Hair extensions must be tightened or removed and replaced every two to six months which increases the chances of damage to your own hair. With clip-in extensions, the ones you snap in and out yourself, damage is less of an issue since weave or glue removal is not required. But clip-ons add weight to your existing hair which can pull it out.

HATS, HELMETS AND HEADBANDS

If hats or helmets are worn for any length of time without cleaning the scalp of oil and perspiration or if a headband is holding oil and perspiration on the top or sides of the scalp, the follicles are getting clogged.

If you wear any kind of headgear or have been perspiring due to exercise, work or sauna, remove the headgear whenever possible and wipe that excess perspiration and oil off the top of your scalp. Be sure to cleanse your scalp as soon as you can.

Women do not appear to have as much perspiration and oil secretions as men do. As a result, the oil or sweat problem is never severe enough for women to go completely bald.

7. LET YOUR HAIR DRY NATURALLY

Whenever you can, let your hair dry naturally. Use a hair dryer on your hair only when you're in a hurry. This will cut down on unnecessary drying out of the hair which causes it to break.

8. HOW TO COMB YOUR HAIR

When combing your wet hair, gently work out the tangles starting at the bottom and work your way up.

Use a wide-toothed comb with rounded edges so your hair doesn't snag. Be very gentle as wet hair can break easily.

9. HOW TO USE CURLING AND FLAT IRONS

During styling, keep those curling and flat irons moving on your hair. Don't hold them in any one place for too long. If you do this the damage is minimal.

An excellent way to protect your hair from the heat of irons is to smooth a tiny amount of apricot kernel oil or some other kind of natural heat-protector product on your hair first.

If you need to hold the curling iron still to get the style you want, I suggest wrapping that section of hair first in hair wraps before applying heat. You can find hair wraps at a beauty-supply store. High heat will, over time, make the hair so dry that the hair will break or split.

10.   CONSUME HIGH-QUALITY PROTEIN

Hair is spun from the protein in the blood. Proteins are made up of amino acids. Amino acids are essential in making hair its thickest and strongest.

Research has determined that a diet lacking in proteins will result in hair becoming brittle, weak and dull, which leads to the increase of broken hair.

Recently I read a story about a woman whose hair had been falling out over a long period of time. When she consumed the proper amount of protein for her body, the hair-loss reduced to normal and her hair got strong.

Consume proteins that sound good to you, whether it's meat, poultry, fish, grains or legumes. Be aware that you can overdo it on the protein. There's agreement among many health professionals that our bodies do best on 15% protein intake in relation to our total diet. Sometimes the requirements are less, sometimes more according to your body type.

Too much protein can cause calcium loss from the bones and cause kidney and liver problems. Protein takes the longest to digest in the stomach making the stomach overwork if protein consumption is too high.

Listen to what your body wants and in the right amount. If you eat meat, ensure it's antibiotic-free and hormone-free. Take enzymes with your proteins, especially meat.

Consume high-quality organic protein in the right amount for your body.

11.   CORRECT NUTRITION AND DIET

Whether we like it or not, hair is an indicator of vitality and overall health. Hair can be made healthier at any age by a proper diet and good nutrition.

High-quality organic protein, whole grains, nuts, fruits, vegetables and herbs are your sources of nutrition.

The herbs rosemary, nettle and horsetail encourage hair growth by promoting blood circulation to the scalp and unclog the pores so nutrients can get to the hair follicles easily. It's important to understand the healing properties and benefits of herbs. The subject of herbs is a whole science in itself so it's best not to take them randomly without consulting a professional educated in herbs.

I cannot in good conscience write a book on hair without covering the subject of nutrition and diet as good nutrition is essential to hair growth. There is a chapter on diet later on that will help remove a lot of confusion on what to eat.

12.   VEGETABLE JUICING

As you read earlier about how my hair grew so long and healthy in such a short period of time—vegetable juices, vegetable juices, vegetable juices! Fresh juices provide *vital,* live vitamins and minerals our bodies *require* for health.

A *variety* of fresh juices supply minerals so lacking in today's diet! I've found that most people are very uninformed on the subject of minerals. Without the right minerals and in the right amounts, *nothing* in the body

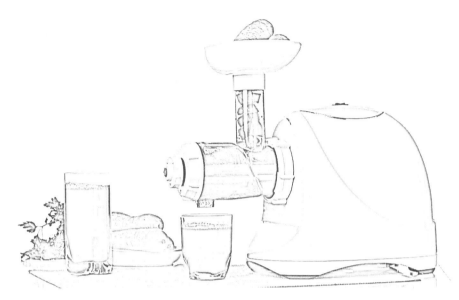

will work properly, including intake of vitamins, as minerals are the basic building blocks. This is *essential* to know and remember.

As an interesting side note, the liver is the largest gland and can regenerate itself if damaged. The liver is the body's detoxifier. It detoxifies harmful substances before they enter the bloodstream and harm the body. All green drinks help detoxify the liver: spinach, kale, parsley, zucchini, dandelion leaves, cucumber, etc. Fresh juices reduce the burden on the liver.

Knowing that, it's important to implement green juices gradually so your body doesn't detoxify too quickly and cause discomfort. You can also dilute the juice to your liking with distilled water.

Note: If green juice isn't tasty to you, you can sweeten it with apple or carrot juice.

Remember, the best, best, best way to have thick, lush hair is vegetable juice, especially carrot juice! I cannot use enough exclamations. Carrot juice, along with the other minerals and vitamins it contains is very high in beta-carotene which produces vitamin A, the vitamin responsible for beautiful hair and skin.

Those people with blood-sugar problems sometimes have difficulty with too much carrot juice, as it is high in natural sugar. If that's the case, monitor the amount of carrot juice you consume or drink green juices only.

Mother Nature has given us a true miracle in carrots and greens. She knows how to make your hair and skin gorgeous.

PROCEDURE FOR JUICING

The combination of carrot, cucumber and celery juice is a good base. Add two to three other ingredients each time: beets, parsley (use only small amounts of these two as they are powerful cleansers), dandelion greens, kale, spinach, lettuce (never iceberg, it has no nutritional value), or whatever sounds good at the time.

If you don't have a juicer, a lot of health food stores make fresh organic juice. You can bring glass canning jars with you and tell them what you want. In the long run it's much less expensive to do your own juicing. If you're truly dedicated to having beautiful, thick hair, you'll want to drink vegetable juice every day.

It is ideal is to drink the juice within 15-20 minutes after being made. After that the vitamins start to dissipate, but the minerals do remain intact.

If you don't have time to juice every day, make enough juice for two to three days. If you choose to do this, put the juice you don't drink that day in small canning jars with vacuum-sealed tops to prevent it from spoiling. Fill the jars all the way to the top so as little air as possible gets into the jar.

See the "Products" section at www.themodernrapunzel.com for different kinds of juicers according to specific needs.

HOW MUCH FRESH JUICE SHOULD BE IN ONE'S DAILY DIET?

That depends on the state of your health.

Here's an eye-opening fact: Hair loss, strictly from the nutritional side of things, comes from the system being too acidic. Acid-forming foods are processed foods, foods not in their whole state. There's a chapter coming up to assist you in getting off junk food that is fun (believe it or not) and works.

So let's do a little defining here without getting too technical. This is very important to understand. "Acid" and "alkaline" are terms that describe one's "pH." pH is a scale that measures how acid or alkaline something is. Alkaline is the opposite of acid.

The blood has to be slightly alkaline for health. On a scale of 1 to 14, below 7 is acid, and above 7 is alkaline; 7 is neutral. Our blood has a pH value of 7.35, which is just slightly alkaline. You can obtain pH urine and saliva strips for testing from most drug stores.

If you consume foods and beverages that are not wholesome and contain "unpronounceable" ingredients not derived directly from Mother Nature as in processed food and soda, the body becomes acidic. Then you are in real trouble because the blood affects *everything*. Ill health and hair loss is due to an over-acidic condition.

Wean off those processed foods and soft drinks until they're completely eliminated from your diet. Shifting the pH from acid to the optimum alkaline range is essential.

You may have heard of people checking the pH of their swimming pool or fish tank. If the fish tank gets too acidic, the fish get sick. An improper pH balance results in ill health for people, too.

Start out gradually with the amount of juice and add a little more each day. Otherwise you'll detoxify too quickly. If you consume juice gradually and then continue to add a little more each week, you'll start to feel better and better and you will start noticing your hair and skin are beginning to look better too.

It's important to be aware of how much juice you need by how much you want. Make combinations of vegetable juice that taste good to you. If it's not sweet enough, add an apple. Believe it or not, some weeks the bitter taste of dandelion green juice tastes great to me.

Pick out vegetables that look and taste good to you, those you naturally gravitate toward. You can also experiment with a variety of others (green, red, yellow, orange and any color vegetables) to see if they suit your taste. Your desires will change. Go with it.

Here's a very beneficial tip: It's best to sip, instead of gulp the juice. Underneath the tongue are openings that go directly into your system. By letting the juice swish around in your mouth before swallowing, you're giving your bloodstream instant access to the healing alkaline juices.

Juicing and eating whole, unprocessed foods will help return the body to the optimum alkaline state. How long that takes depends on how acidic your system is. It takes less time to return the body to health than it did to abuse it, but it will take as long as it takes for each individual person. It's the minerals in vegetable juices that return the body to the alkaline state.

Your body must have the minerals contained in fresh juices and pure organic foods to grow new hair.

Drink a *variety* of your fresh-made, mineral-abundant vegetable juices!

13.   PABA, PANOTHENIC ACID AND B VITAMINS

PABA (Para-Amino Benzoic Acid) prevents the hair from graying and retards hair loss. Panothenic Acid has also been shown to be very effective in correcting hair loss.

The entire B Complex vitamin is a must to stop hair loss and restore a full head of hair. B vitamins are depleted during times of stress. The more stress one is experiencing, the higher dose or frequency is required.

14.   HORMONES

After age 30 and sometimes even in the 20's, one can experience hair loss due to low hormone levels. As hormone levels decline, less nutrition and oxygen gets to the hair root. Over time, low hormone levels can cause the re-growth stage to slow down and, a horrifying thought, eventually stop.

Some of the other symptoms stemming from lack of hormones in addition to hair loss include depression, nervousness, mood swings, irritability, feeling hopeless, excessive worry, suicidal thoughts, crying easily, aging, chronic fatigue, exhaustion, headaches, weight gain, lowered immune system, bone loss, high and low blood pressure and trouble with sleep, mental fog, mental confusion, poor concentration, forgetfulness, to name a few.

There is a great deal of controversy about hormones: whether to take them or not, creams or oral, etc., etc. I recommend you do your own research and have your hormone levels tested. Gather enough information to find what works for you. I have found what works for me but each woman is different.

Here is some information from Dr. Ian Shillington regarding hormones. He says,

"Nowadays, the subject of hormones is almost as popular as a coyote in a chicken coop. There's PMS, menopause difficulties, infertility, hair loss plus many other conditions too numerous to mention.

"A major CAUSE of ALL of these problems is the amount of hormones, steroids and antibiotics used in the entire commercial meat industry! You and your family should eat ORGANIC meats only!"

He goes on to say,

"The best approach is to find the true 'cause' [of hormonal imbalance] and then correct the vitamin, mineral, nutritional and biochemical imbalances, thus allowing the body to once again stabilize its own hormones. Once you find the 'Cause' you can then stop doing those things that created the imbalance in the first place."

There are effective herbs and herbal tinctures which help put the hormones under control until one's system can balance out through correct supplementation and nutrition as mentioned by Dr. Shillington. Consult your doctor, holistic physician or natural health-care practitioner.

See Dr. Shillington's herbal tinctures at OrganicSolutionsStore.com or contact his office at: Office@AcademyOfNaturalHealing.com for a free copy of his audio lecture on handling these things *naturally*.

Do you want to be and stay young? Having your hormones balanced keeps the blues and much, much more away!

You don't need to suffer. You deserve to be the sensual, delicious woman you are, your whole life!

15.   LOW ADRENALS

Female hair loss can be linked to the adrenal glands. Low adrenal levels have been attributed to lack of sleep, poor nutrition and too much stress. There are sections on each of these coming up.

It is important to know that the adrenal glands produce estrogen, progesterone, DHEA and other hormones. Therefore if the adrenals are weak, they can have a difficult time producing essential hormones.

Who knows how many hormone problems actually stem from low adrenals?

It is also important to know that if one is chronically tired due to adrenal exhaustion the answer is not caffeine. Caffeine is a stimulant that can wear out the adrenals and eventually the adrenals are so tired that even caffeine has no effect.

To correct this situation, one needs to rebuild the system through balancing body chemistry and providing essential nutrients. Have your adrenal function checked by a natural health-care practitioner.

Women with thinning hair due to low adrenal function can benefit from using herbs such as Siberian ginseng, astragalus and licorice root. If you decide to take any of these herbs, please consult with your natural health-care professional first. Caution: Licorice root should not be used if you're pregnant or have high blood pressure.

If you have been experiencing chronic exhaustion, email me and I will send you a link to an article written by a brilliant doctor on how to address this area fully.

16.   THYROID DIFFICULTIES

In some cases you will need to do a blood test to see where your thyroid levels are. Your levels may be hypo = too low, or hyper = too high or both, believe it or not. A competent doctor or natural health practitioner will put you on the correct supplement or medicine to correct it. Natural health practitioners also test thyroid levels through something called Applied Kinesiology.

17.   TOXINS

A toxic body can cause hair loss. When a body is coping with too many poisons, it's difficult for it to be able to function properly. See the section coming up on the toxic load and detoxification.

18.   STRESS

Stress is said to be one of the leading causes of hair loss, if not the leading. See Chapter 13: "The Factors of Stress and Hair Loss."

You have just read a lot of information. To help make it easy, in the back of the book are charts outlining what specific procedures to implement according to the condition of your hair. Remember, it is important to review what you just read enough times so that you have all the details as the chart itself cannot cover them all.

I hope these 18 potential causes of hair loss and their solutions have helped educate, enlighten and inspire you to bring about the gorgeous head of hair you want!

Let me re-cap all 18 of them:

1. Magic Overnight Hair Beautification
2. Get rid of split ends
3. Brushing and massage
4. Free up congestion in the scalp
5. Limit chemical processing and avoid using chemical hair products
6. Do your best to eliminate hair restraints
7. If possible, let your hair dry naturally
8. While combing your wet hair, gently work out the tangles by starting at the bottom and working up
9. Keep curling-irons and flat-irons moving
10. Consume high-quality protein
11. Correct nutrition and diet (See Chapters 10 and 11)
12. Vegetable juicing
13. PABA and Pantothenic Acid—See your nutritionist for amounts
14. Hormones—See your natural health-care practitioner
15. Low adrenals—See your natural health-care practitioner
16. Thyroid—See a competent health-care practitioner
17. Toxins (See Chapter 12)
18. Stress (See Chapter 13)

Most of the procedures written in this chapter will make a difference now and others over time. Be patient. Continue.

Let's now take up the rest of the factors that will encourage even greater results!

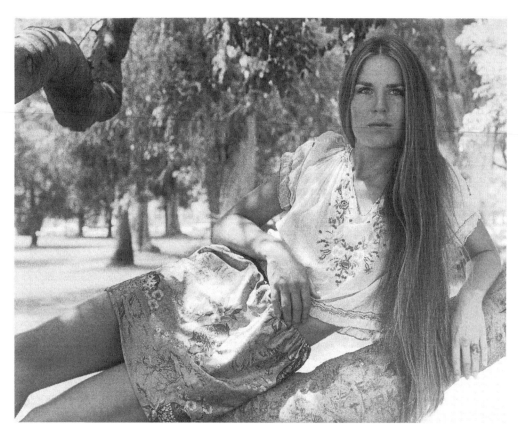

1973 – Los Angeles

Chapter Five

How to Help Your Hair

hat about other problems we can experience with our hair besides hair loss? Hair can need help in other ways. This chapter provides remedies I have found to be effective in correcting additional problems with our hair.

These areas are: how to help hair that isn't growing fast enough to get it to the length you want, how to prevent your hair from breaking, drying and graying and what to do about dandruff and itchy scalp. Also included are some fun tricks for long hair.

I hope you find these solutions as useful as I have.

How to Help Your Hair Grow Longer

How many women are resorting to hair extensions to have the look of longer hair? A lot!

As hair gets longer, the cuticle (outside layer) starts to wear away, leaving hair susceptible to damage and breakage. The cuticle is extremely important to the condition of the hair because of its protective functions.

Cuticle damage is caused by abuse during styling and by chemical products. Bobby pins, barrettes or any kind of hair restraints may cause damage to the cuticle. High heat from blow dryers, flat irons, and hot rollers can weaken the hair, leading to split ends which cause the hairs to break off. High water pressure and even moderately hot water will cause the cuticle to peel. Abuse, such as brushing the hair while wet and not combing the tangles out gently may cause extreme damage to the hair that can be nearly impossible to repair.

IF YOU WANT LONGER HAIR:

   a. Cut off all split ends.
   b. Follow the three-step Magic Overnight Beautification Process: 1) use a chlorine shower filter, 2) clarify your hair and, 3) apply oil(s) to the hair.
   c. Use chemical-free hair products.
   d. Drink your vegetable juices.
   e. Use moderate water pressure while rinsing your hair.
   f. Use warm water only on your hair while rinsing, never hot.
   g. Use a wide-toothed comb to gently comb out wet hair, starting from the bottom and working up.
   h. Let your hair dry naturally whenever possible.
   i. Brush your hair only when it's completely dry.
   j. Keep your curling and flat irons moving while you're styling and/or protect your hair from the heat with wraps obtained from a beauty supply store.
   k. Eliminate bobby pins and barrettes and anything else that may pinch your hair or hold it in one position for any length of time.
   l. See the section on slant boards for the scalp massage technique.
   m. See the next two sections on how to help handle breakage and dryness.

How to Prevent Your Hair from Breaking

   1. Never use friction (brisk rubbing) while drying your hair with the towel. After shampooing and conditioning and while still in the shower, squeeze the excess water out of your hair. Then use the towel as a turban to soak up moisture.

Do not "dry" your hair by rubbing it back and forth with a towel.

2. Always use a wide-toothed comb to detangle wet hair. Always! And comb it out starting from the bottom up, gradually taking out tangles as you go. You will have little to no tangles if your hair has been conditioned well.

3. Let your hair dry naturally whenever possible. Heat from a hair dryer damages the cuticle of the hair. If you need to use a hair dryer on an on-going basis, use it on warm, never hot.

4. Brush your hair only when it's completely dry. Use a good brush that has widely-spaced bristles and rounded ends. If it snags, throw it away and get another one. A very good natural brush is boar bristle.

5. Always keep your curling or flat-iron moving while you're styling or use wraps to protect your hair from the heat. Wraps are obtained from a beauty supply store.

6. Eliminate bobby pins and barrettes and anything else that may pinch your hair or hold it in one position for a long time.

7. For curly hair, condition your hair in the shower, and then while you're still in the shower or when you first get out, use a wide-toothed pick to comb it. Let it dry naturally and then, if you need to, use a natural gel for styling and dimension.

How to Prevent Dryness

1. Use the Three-Step Magic Overnight Beautification Process.

2. I'm sure you've heard a million times not to wash your hair frequently if it's dry. Well, it's true. Wash it only when you have to. But don't despair, using the oils I mentioned will change the condition of dryness and soon you'll be able to wash it more frequently.

3. The crisis handling for dry ends before they split and have to be cut off is: Put about a teaspoon of jojoba oil (castor oil if your ends are exceptionally dry) and vitamin E on one of your palms and mix the two together. Saturate the dry ends of your hair with this mixture and leave it on for half an

hour to an hour. Be gentle when you wash it out. It works like magic for dry ends!

4. When your hair is frizzy, it needs moisture. Take a very small amount of apricot kernel or coconut oil, spread it on your hands and then very lightly coat the outside surface of your hair with your hands. It gives the hair shine, smoothness and gets rid of "the frizzies."

5. If your hair is long, a good way to condition it and give it a fabulous shine for the next day is to braid it loosely before you go to bed. Use snag-free rubber bands to bind it at the ends.

6. Essential fatty acids taken internally known as "EFA's" are exactly that; Essential Fatty Acids,; essential for health. They are: omega 3, 6, and 9.

Take these fresh oils in capsules from your health food store. The amount to take is on the bottle.

Have you noticed the quality of your pet's coat when oil is added to the diet? It glistens! It's the same for your hair.

7. Last but not least are the techniques mentioned earlier of: a) taking saunas with oil in your hair, b) using an old-fashioned hair dryer with a hood with oil in your hair and, c) putting oil in your hair for a half hour to an hour before you shampoo.

How to Help Reverse and Prevent Graying

1. Gray hair is mostly a mineral deficiency. It can also be genetic. It can also be brought on by stress.

In my early 50's my hair started to gray. I thought it was genetic because my mother's hair starting graying in her 50's also. So I started doing what everyone else does. I started covering it up.

But one day, seemingly all of a sudden, when it was time to color my roots, I noticed something very interesting. While looking closely at how much coloring needed to be done, I noticed that I had very little gray hair; maybe 5% compared to over 25% a month or two earlier.

What happened? What did I do that was different? The only thing I did differently was that I had resumed vegetable juicing after not juicing for some time. So over the next few months, I watched my "graying" closely.

Since then I rarely go a day without vegetable juice. I have a few silver hairs here and there and minimal graying as long as I continue to juice.

So much for genetics. I'm not saying your hair won't turn gray due to genetics but mine was not caused by it. Perhaps yours isn't either. Along with my own experience, I've had readers who have reported their graying significantly diminish by drinking fresh, mineral-abundant vegetable juices.

Drinking fresh vegetable juices is invaluable, not just for the hair but for all the other countless health benefits. There are wonderful books on juicing which give the recipes to follow for every type of health situation.

2. Powdered products abundant with dried greens and just about everything a body needs nutritionally are available. If you're on the go and can't drink your fresh juice every day, these are great. These dried greens are a great source of minerals for graying hair. Remember the man who grew his hair back in six months? Along with applying castor oil to his scalp, he consumed dried greens daily. They supply essential nutrition and are a great way to give one's body what it needs easily and quickly.

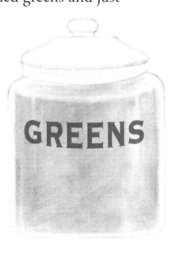

See the "Products" section at www.themodernrapunzel.com for an excellent product with dried greens.

3. Para-Amino Benzoic Acid (PABA) has been known to prevent hair from graying.

4. The B vitamin Biotin is known to prevent graying. Vitamin B Complex has been called the "hair vitamin." A deficiency in this vitamin is caused by stress in any form. It's absolutely vital B vitamin deficiencies are handled. They are key to hair growth.

One expert has said it's best to take vitamin B and Biotin before going to bed and the other vitamins and minerals in the morning. Some people say B vitamins keep them awake at night and some say it helps them sleep better. You'll have to do your own experimenting.

5. Stress, again! Who lives without stress in this world with the exception of...wow, I can't think of anyone!

Stress has been known to be one of the leading causes of graying hair, if not *the* leading. It is essential to know how to manage stress in the course of daily living.

Please take what you learn in the upcoming section on stress to heart as it's vital for the health of your hair and overall well-being.

The physical and mental affect each other, positively or negatively. When a person feels and looks better physically, it will help one feel better mentally also, and vice versa.

That gray just might go away with good nutrition and lowered stress.

What to Do About Dandruff

Per a cosmetologist, dandruff is caused by excess oil secreted from the follicle mixing with the dead flakes the skin sheds from the scalp.

Dandruff shampoo obviously cannot prevent the scalp from shedding skin or the follicle from secreting oil. It only places a barrier between the two. That barrier clogs the follicles of the scalp which leads to more hair loss.

It's next to impossible to get a regular dandruff shampoo that eliminates the real cause or without chemicals.

Use a massager on your scalp and/or do the massage technique without oil described in the section on slant boards until the oil glands are functioning normally. I've found this helps handle dandruff more effectively than anything else.

Discontinue consuming fried and fatty foods. Don't wear anything on your head that would have a tendency to hold excess oil to your scalp as in hats, helmets, wigs or headbands. Use only oil-free shampoos and conditioners.

What to Do About Itchy Scalp

An itchy scalp is mostly due to dry scalp, clogged follicles or a minor scalp infection.

REMEDIES I'VE FOUND TO HELP ITCHY SCALP:
1. More people than one would suppose have itchy scalps as a result of running their fingers through their hair. The only

explanation for that would be their hands are not clean enough at the time and carry bacteria.

If you have a tendency to run your hands through your hair, make sure your hands are squeaky clean. Try this first and if it is not the cause, try one or more of the remedies listed below.

2. If itchy scalp is due to dryness, jojoba oil gently rubbed into the scalp for a couple minutes may help. Make sure you shampoo immediately afterwards.

3. Itching can be from clogged follicles or new hair trying to break through. Gentle use of a massager on the scalp oftentimes brings relief as you're assisting the follicles to open. If that doesn't do it, the use of a chemical-free follicle cleanser can oftentimes eliminate itching completely.

4. If your scalp is oily and itches, the use of a massager will help normalize the excess oil secretions from the follicles thus helping to reduce or eliminate the itchiness.

5. A shampoo from your health food store containing any or all of these ingredients: tea tree oil, neem oil, MSM, rosewood oil, colloidal silver and rosemary are effective. Use tea tree and neem oil sparingly as they can, over time, clog the follicles. I found a very good natural shampoo with tea tree oil that works great.

6. Remember to take essential fatty acids internally. They make a big difference in how lubricated your scalp and skin are. The body needs to be lubricated from the inside as well as out with healthy oils.

It's much easier to take EFA's in capsules rather than liquid as the taste is not very pleasant, but some brave souls can withstand it. Either way, liquid or capsule, make sure it's in the refrigerated section of your health-food store or hasn't been sitting on the shelf for long as it can go rancid.

7. Aloe vera gel. The gel of the aloe vera plant is amazing for its healing properties. If your scalp has a rash or itchiness that just doesn't seem to go away, aloe vera might just be the answer.

There are some juicers sturdy enough to extract the gel out of the aloe vera plant but not many. Pure aloe vera gel is available in the health-food store. Make sure you get the gel for this purpose, not the juice. You can also find an aloe vera gel with neem oil in it that works well for itchiness.

Aloe vera helps heal everything from sunburns to upset stomach to rashes and much, much more. It should be in everyone's refrigerator. Along with its healing properties, it contains vital minerals the hair and body needs.

8. Itchy scalp can be from the scalp being exposed to bright sun for an extended time. In that case, wear a hat during the height of the day when the sun is beating down. Make sure you wash any perspiration from your scalp.

9. Once in a while an itchy scalp can be due to a scalp infection. Your natural health practitioner might recommend adding a few drops of tea tree oil or colloidal silver to your shampoo as a natural remedy.

I suggest using a massager and refrain from running your fingers through your hair first. If that doesn't handle the problem, find a shampoo with one or more of the above natural ingredients obtainable at your health-food store. You can buy one or more of the ingredients separately and then combine your shampoo and the item you chose in the palm of your hand, one shampooing at a time until you find the one that works the best for you.

To recap:

1. Keep your hands clean if you have the habit of running your fingers through your hair.

2. Gently rub jojoba oil into the scalp for a couple minutes and then wash out.

3. Use a massager gently on your scalp. Use an all-natural follicle cleanser.

4. Use a massager if your scalp is oily.

5. Use a shampoo from your health food store containing one or more of the listed ingredients.

6. Take Essential Fatty Acids internally.

7. Apply Aloe Vera gel by itself or Aloe with Neem oil on the scalp.

8. Wear a hat when out in the sun.

9. If you have a scalp infection, try using one or more of the ingredients listed in #5 above in your shampoo until you

find the one that works for you or see your natural health practitioner.

One or more of the nine suggestions should help remedy the situation. It has for me. I used to be bothered with itchy scalp and now I know exactly what to do.

Three Tricks for Long Hair

TO MAKE YOUR HAIR LOOK FULLER

1. Whenever you can, let your hair air-dry. And then when it's just a little damp, blow-dry it upside-down on low setting until it's completely dry. Wait at least five minutes for your hair to fully cool and settle down before you brush or comb it as the heat from drying makes it very vulnerable to breakage. Once it's dry gently brush it right-side up until the tangles are gone.

Now turn your head upside-down again and brush your hair forward starting from the back of your neck. Continue the process of gently brushing your entire head upside-down until you can feel the circulation throughout your whole scalp. This takes only a minute.

After you've done that and before turning right-side up again, take a cloth ponytail holder and secure your hair at the top of your head. Turn right-side up. Wait 10-15 minutes, take the holder out and let it settle on its own. This will give wonderful fullness to the top of the hair.

TO CREATE WAVES FOR LONG HAIR

2. When your hair is a tiny bit damp, twist it from the back as tight as you need for the wave you want and use a clip to hold it. Wait for a half hour to an hour until your hair is dry and then release your hair from the clip. Your hair will be very shiny as the hair shaft has calmed down and you'll have soft, lovely waves.

3. Sometimes after my hair is washed and a tiny bit wet, I put ten or so loose braids in my hair and secure the ends with

very small non-snag rubber bands. I sleep on them and wake up in the morning with soft, smooth waves.

Chapter Six

No-Nos and Yes-Yeses

No-Nos

If you're a swimmer, you're especially aware of the damage chlorine causes hair. I knew a swimmer whose hair turned green from swimming in a chlorine pool.

A trick you can use to prevent chlorine damage is: saturate your hair with a thick oil, like olive oil, especially around the front hairline, and then put a tight swim cap on, concentrating the oil especially where water might seep in.

The best solution of all is to swim in the ocean or a lake instead of a chlorine pool. Salt-water pools are becoming more and more popular.

PARABEN PRESERVATIVES

Exactly what are paraben preservatives? Per "Paraben Preservatives and Cosmetics: Controversy and Alternatives" written by Adams Kristin,

> "Parabens are found in approximately 75-90% of cosmetics such as make-up, lotion, deodorants and shampoos. According to 'A Consumers Dictionary of Cosmetic Ingredients', water is the only cosmetic ingredient used more frequently than paraben preservatives.

Increasing concern for the safety of ingredients in cosmetics has brought some widely-used cosmetic preservatives by the family name 'paraben' to center stage. Paraben preservatives are listed under multiple names and are used to preserve the majority of cosmetics on the market today...

According to recent research, more than 60 percent of topically applied chemicals via cosmetics, lotions, etc. are absorbed by the skin and dispersed throughout the body by the bloodstream. Once absorbed into the body, paraben preservatives mimic the hormone estrogen and can disrupt the body's normal hormonal balance."

Any time hormones are disrupted, there is the liability of hair loss, depression, anxiety, mental confusion, memory loss and a multitude of other problems.

Any product labels you see with "paraben" or "para-", stay away from them!

Two other chemicals commonly found in hair products are sodium laurel sulfate, which has been found to be a cause of hair loss, and cetyl alcohol which dries out the hair. Stay away also from any product with an ingredient labeled "propyl-".

Look at the labels of the products you use or are considering buying and do your own research on the effects of that chemical before you use it.

Of the thousands of chemicals used in body-care products, only a small percentage has been tested for toxicity. This is a global health crisis. These chemicals are ingested into our bodies and washed into our waters every day. The less we use, the less our bodies and waters suffer from unnecessary pollution. Do your absolute best to eliminate them altogether by using only natural products.

"Natural" means something found the way it is in nature. We don't have to suffer the long list of ills due to these toxic substances. The safest thing to do, for yourself, your loved ones and the planet, is to use only those products free of toxic chemicals.

Yes-Yeses

In my experience I've found that alternating shampoos and conditioners makes my hair much healthier and stronger.

Each product contains different nutrients for the hair and as a result gives the hair more life and fullness because the hair is getting a wide variety of natural substances. I have four to five chemical-free, natural shampoos and three to four conditioners on hand at all times.

You'll notice a big difference in the health of your hair when you do this.

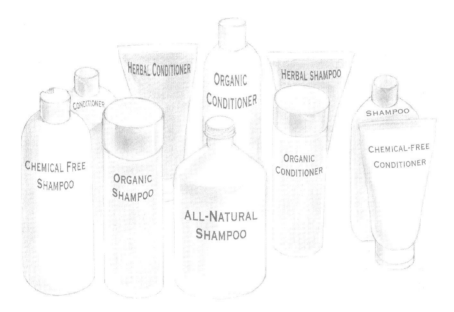

As mentioned earlier, use only warm water, never hot, on your hair. Shampoo and condition, rinse with warm water and then gradually and comfortably make the water cool to cold for the final rinse. This closes the hair shaft, making the hair smoother and less frizzy when it's dry. Most importantly, it stimulates the scalp by waking it up.

Who knows how much new hair comes in from just this one activity!

Chapter Seven

Slant Boards

The Most Vital Piece of Equipment You'll Ever Own for Your Hair and Whole Body

Slant boards!

Here is the long-awaited section on slant boards. A slant board is, in my opinion and experience, the most health-giving piece of equipment you can own and use. The benefits are vast. What you are about to read is very enlightening.

To quote Larry Jacobs, an expert on slanting and author of the book Standing up to Gravity: How to Fight the Law and Win,

"We can't see Gravity. We can't hear Gravity. Nor can we touch, taste or smell Gravity. Thus, when it comes to keeping up our health and beauty, we seldom think about Gravity and its powerful influence over our mental and physical well-being in our earth-bound lives. Yet, the effects of Gravity's constant downward pull on our faces, necks, shoulders, chests, backs, organs, hips, legs and feet are painfully obvious to most of us. For instance, it's not old age which causes our bodies to shrink on this planet: it's Gravity!

If Gravity can prevent water from flowing upward, it can also prevent the blood in our bodies from flowing upward freely (above our hearts) and into our heads—whenever we sit, stand and sleep with our heads on top of pillows. And poor blood circulation up to our eyes, ears, gums, faces, scalps and brains is a good reason why these, our most precious faculties, deteriorate first during our earthly existence. For most of us, simply sitting and standing can be a never-ending uphill battle against Gravity. And, whether we realize it or not, the longer we maintain these positions, the more of our human energy is drained by Gravity.

The heavy hand of Gravity also takes its toll on our internal organs. It compresses our lungs and limits breathing capacity; it prolapses our colons and slows metabolism and elimination. Gravity makes the ground rule! It's the law of the land! And we're stuck to this planet because of it. In short, no upright person escapes its endless downsizing of the human body. Bottomline: Every aspect of our well-grounded existence is undermined by Gravity.

Slant boards have been popular in the natural health and beauty industry for many years. It's a lazy way to perk up your youth and vitality. If inverting your body is a topsy-turvy concept to you, you may wish to seek the advice of a wellness expert before you begin. But you can't escape Gravity's pitfalls on this planet."

Who would have ever thought the influence of gravity would play such a major role in our health and well-being?

Slant boards reverse the earth's continuous gravitational pull on the body by lying with the head lower than the feet by 17 inches. As a result of this reversal, circulation is increased to the scalp. Nutrition can then flow to the follicles—*nutrition vital in growing new hair.*

Through slanting, the organs and muscles throughout the entire body also heal and strengthen.

For example, many women experience partial loss of bladder control. Like every other organ, the bladder is being pulled down by gravity. And because the bladder holds fluid, it has more weight and can be affected by gravity even more. Reversing the gravitational pull helps strengthen those muscles and gives the bladder a break from the constant strain.

Not only are you giving the bladder and every other organ relief by relaxing them, they now have a chance to regain their resiliency and strength.

The benefits go on and on. As Larry said, "It's not old age which causes our bodies to shrink on this planet: it's Gravity!"

Slanting is the ideal time to give yourself a scalp massage. Again, massage on a slant board facilitates the replacement of old blood with new life-giving blood and as long as you're eating well, nourishment is then fed to the hair follicles, whereas before they were being starved.

The correct method of giving oneself a scalp massage makes an enormous difference. Do not underestimate the power and effectiveness of this. It is directly related to improving the health of the scalp, how fast hair grows and new hair-growth.

SCALP MASSAGE

First, a little important education:

Every hair on your head has two basic parts—the hair follicle and the hair shaft. The follicle is where the hair grows from. Each follicle flows with tiny blood vessels. Follicles are connected to a sebaceous gland, which provides the hair with a protective natural oil called sebum. When you stimulate the scalp through massage, the follicles release that protective oil, blood can flow and the follicles open up and get nourished. Then new hair can form and break through.

I know from personal experience that hairs can become trapped in the follicles underneath the scalp, hairs that were not able to break through because the follicles were clogged. I've had hair pop out of my scalp one to two inches and longer as a result of proper massage and cleansing. It occurs the more the procedures are closely followed.

Those previously trapped hairs that have broken through have a different look. They can tend to look "corkscrew" and are generally thicker than new hair. When your hair is dry, sometimes you can see them. They stick up. It's fun to see them appear.

Generally new hair is finer. They're a little harder to see but they're there.

You can well imagine what would happen if the right kind of massage was done on the scalp to allow existing and new hairs to break through.

You can give yourself a scalp massage with or without jojoba or castor oil. If you want to help handle thinning and bald spots, this is the right time to use oil; while slanting.

HOW TO DO A SCALP MASSAGE WITH OIL WHILE SLANTING:

a. Place a very small amount of either jojoba or castor oil onto the thinning parts of your scalp. (If you like, this is also an opportune time to put jojoba oil through your hair for your weekly oil treatment).

b. With the tips of your fingers of both hands placed on the back of your neck, one set of fingers on each side, gently move your fingers in a circular motion. (In other words, don't rub or move your fingers back and forth or up and down. Keep them firmly and comfortably on your scalp while moving your fingers in a circular motion.)

c. Continue this exact motion with your fingers up and around your whole scalp, ending up on the top. You may find some sore spots and ridges. Gently but firmly massage those spots, but not too much at one time.

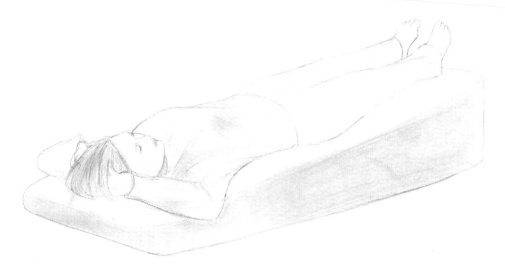

d. This whole procedure should take about five minutes. You don't just want to focus on the areas that are thin or thinning. To grow new hair you need circulation throughout your whole scalp.

e. Carefully shampoo your scalp with a chemical-free and oil-free shampoo to remove the oil. You can plan your oil scalp massage on the days you regularly wash your hair.

f. When you're done washing your hair and it's dry, use a massager for a minute or so to help any trapped hairs break through.

My suggestion in starting out is to do this procedure once a week. This gives your scalp the chance to get used to the oil and increased circulation. After two or more weeks, you can increase the oil massage to two times a week depending on how quickly hairs are breaking through the follicles with once a week. If the hair is breaking through just fine, continue with once a week. Don't change anything.

In other words, increase the oil massage to two times a week if you're not seeing hair pop out of the follicles with once a week.

No matter what, for anyone, it's a good idea to do this procedure once a week to keep the follicles free of congestion.

As I mentioned earlier, castor oil is very thick and jojoba oil is lighter. If the scalp has been balding for some time, castor oil is recommended.

DAILY USE OF THE SLANT BOARD WITHOUT OILS

In addition to your scalp massage with oil once a week, use of the slant board, with or without oil massage, relaxes the cranial area (the head) and opens up the blood flow to the entire scalp. Massage, while slanting, relieves tension and allows the scalp to move easily and fluidly over the skull.

Lying on a slant board with a 17 inch incline, even with no massage, will bring circulation to the scalp through reversing gravity. The scalp is getting the blood supply and nutrition it so desperately needs. Massage helps it along faster.

It's very refreshing to lie on a slant board daily even if you don't massage your scalp.

To recap, while slanting:

1. Massage your scalp with oil once a week,
2. massage your scalp without oil the other six days, or
3. just lay on the slant board and relax. It's up to you whether you want to just relax or massage your scalp. You'll get great benefit from both.

Just know relaxation and gentleness is key with all three: massage with oil, massage without oil, or no massage at all on the slant board.

For a short time as you massage your scalp, you may notice a little more hair falling out than usual. This is not a bad thing and there's no need to be alarmed. Those hairs were ready to come out anyway. They need to come out so new healthier ones can come in.

Let me draw an analogy here:

We know that if dying branches and leaves are left on a tree or bush, it will rob the plant of life. One of the inherent characteristics of Nature is that it will try to heal and revive whenever it can. The source of energy that is giving the plant strength will, to some degree, attempt to revive the dying branches and leaves, which of course will rob the healthy plant of some of its power and make the plant less likely to be lush and abundant.

So when the lifeless matter is removed the plant goes, "Oh Boy! Let's grow some new leaves!" Then you don't have to keep fertilizing, watering and pleading with it to survive because its innate life source is not being robbed; only strengthened through removing the drain of its power.

And before you know it, a whole forest is growing out of your scalp! I think you got the idea; unhealthy hair is being replaced by new, healthy hair.

Using the massage procedure as outlined here will not only provide relief from physical stress but will give those follicles a chance to become unplugged so existing or new hair can break through.

For added relaxation and benefit, each time you're done massaging the scalp and while still on the slant board, you can massage your face, too. Use any one of the recommended oils for the hair on your face (except castor oil as it's too thick) so you don't stretch your skin. If your skin is especially dry, I recommend extra virgin olive, avocado or almond oil.

Apply the oil to your face. Then starting from the back of the neck, gently move the tips of your fingers in a circular motion up to the chin, around the ears, to the cheeks and around the eyes to the forehead. When you massage your cheeks and around your eyes, move your fingers outwards from the nose toward your temples, not inwards.

This massage helps drain the lymphatic system of toxins and can help make your face look years younger. It's quite something.

Once done with the scalp and face massage, lying on a slant board for another fifteen to thirty minutes is a wonderful way to relax and rejuvenate. In that short amount of time it can sometimes feel as if one has had a one to two hour nap. With this procedure not only are you resting, but the body is getting strengthened at the same time. There's no other "exercise" that accomplishes what a slant board does. Because it's so easy you may not notice the vast benefits, but it's definitely happening.

Have a slant board that is safe and comfortable with a seventeen-inch incline. A steeper slant board is not needed as you want to gently circulate the blood while reversing gravity. Gentle in anything is always better. When getting up off a lower slant board, one doesn't generally experience the dizziness one can on steeper boards. Turn onto your right side before rising from your slant board and lift your body slowly.

A home-made slant board can be made out of wood or another strong material. If you build one yourself or have one built, use padding and material to make it comfortable. Make sure it's strong, safe and long and wide enough to comfortably fit the whole body.

My two favorite slant boards are an air slant board or one made out of durable long-lasting foam. The air slant boards are portable, light and have a built-in air pump. The foam ones can be folded up after use to be used as a cushion or laid flat for use as a small bed.

See the "Products" section at www.themodernrapunzel.com for comfortable, safe air and foam slant boards.

Now that we've gone over the natural ways to grow a thick, healthy head of hair, let's look at the cost of hair transplant surgery. The minimum cost for a hair transplant is $4,000. The cost of an effective shower filter is about $90, jojoba oil is about $10, a good juicer is around $250, a slant board is anywhere from $69 to $200. Let's just say the overall cost of the natural route is around $500.

What are the other costs of transplant surgery in terms of one's overall well-being versus the procedures outlined here that not only grow hair back naturally, but help restore and ensure one's health for a lifetime?

I'll let you answer that for yourself.

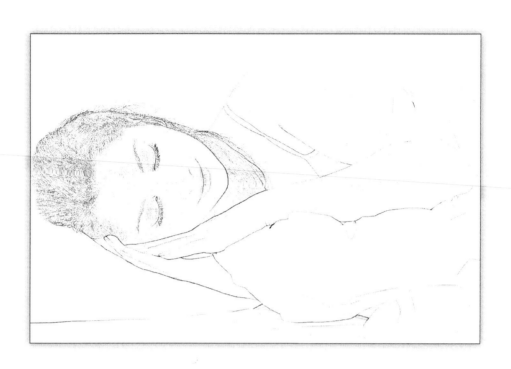

Chapter Eight

Beauty Sleep: The Great Rejuvenator

W hat does sleep have to do with growing a beautiful head of hair? Everything! Here's how:

Sleep is the Great Healer. Sleep is when the whole body replenishes and rejuvenates. When one's body is rejuvenated, one's entire system can grow new cells and that includes new cells for hair growth.

The biggest complaint of Americans is, "I'm tired."

How many times have you heard others proudly say, "I'm a hero! I only sleep five hours a night!," with dark circles, colorless sagging skin, no shine to their hair and bent over because it's too much energy to stand up straight?

Trying to prove something by not getting enough sleep is silly. It is *not heroic or efficient* to work long hours in spite of tiredness. It's self-defeating. One can accomplish at least twice as much when one is rested.

Insufficient sleep reduces our ability to cope with life. Vince Lombardi once made a very wise statement, "Fatigue makes cowards of us all."

Sleep is when *you* rejuvenate. When needed, sleep is The Great Escape. The father of a friend of mine, after a very long and intense work schedule, used to sleep for almost three days straight. There's nothing wrong with that once in awhile. His wife would leave food outside the door. When he awoke, he was a new man; refreshed and confident.

So, get the sleep you need to feel truly rested. Not just "enough." Get the amount you need to operate at *full speed*, whether it's three hours a night or ten. When I need eleven hours sleep, I take it. It rarely happens but the test of its workability is how I feel the next day. It's like having a new life. I then get so much more done and everyone around me is happier because I am.

Let's get real. Our bodies cannot operate for very long with insufficient high-quality sleep without it taking a major toll on one's personal sanity and the well-being of those around us.

Dr. Lawrence Wilson says: "All illnesses start with fatigue." Quite an awakening statement wouldn't you say?

Learn your own sleep deprivation signals. Note what they are as you recognize them. Then take action to remedy them long before you get so exhausted you're not able to function at your normal speed. This could include getting to bed earlier or wearing ear plugs to dampen environmental noise. Take control of whatever is making it difficult to get a deep night's sleep.

Don't try to operate past tiredness or exhaustion. You'll steal from the next day, your life and your courage.

Go to bed.

TIPS FOR THE BEST NIGHT'S SLEEP

I've heard that every hour the body sleeps before midnight is equal to two. It has to do with where the sun is in the heavens in relation to Earth.

Do your best to get to sleep well before midnight.

Black-out curtains in your bedroom helps you sleep like a baby. Sleep on 100% cotton sheets. You'll sleep the deepest. Whenever possible, sleep with your window open to allow fresh air in. Try to have little to no electronics in your bedroom: TV, computer, electric alarm clock, etc. Some people unplug every electrical device before going to sleep as then there are no electro-magnetic frequencies aloft in the space to interfere with one's own energy field. If it's not possible to do that, you can purchase a product to wear around your neck which deflects the energy fields away from your body.

The best beds by far are air mattresses as they have no metal in them. Get a plush one for sleeping every night, not the kind for camping. They can be inflated or deflated according to your desired firmness. They range from $150 to $1,500, depending on how fancy you want to go.

Most air beds, as they are made out of synthetics, need to be aired outside sometimes for as long as two weeks or longer before use. Some of the more expensive air beds are made out of more natural materials and don't need to be aired out as long.

Either an air mattress or a bed set that has no metal will give the best night's sleep. Avoid putting a box spring under the air mattress as the metal coils in the box springs interferes with your own energy field. You can purchase or have a smooth wood platform made to your desired height to place your air mattress on. You'll notice a big difference when you sleep with no metal under your body.

Being *well* rested dramatically helps create a harmonious rhythm in your life for yourself and those around you.

What is that worth? A lot.

Chapter Nine

Water
The Miracle of Nature!

The majority of Americans are chronically dehydrated. This could very likely apply to a large percentage of the world's population.

"Dehydrated" means not enough water.

It's a very interesting fact that 80% of our bodies are made up of water (the other 20% is mineral). What do you think happens if the body doesn't have the water it needs to replace what it eliminates and do its job of cleansing and rejuvenating? The answer is, everything is adversely affected in the body–from the cells to the tissues to the muscles to the internal organs to the skin. *They shrink if not given water and that includes the cells that grow hair!*

Inadequate water results in fatigue and general body aches. The body is thirsty and begging for water, not soft drinks, not coffee, not juice, etc. Water.

Water is required by every function in the body. Water helps clear the body of waste material, it helps fight constipation, aids digestion and cell function, helps lubricate joints, is an important solvent in the body and helps control body temperature.

If your body feels hot and you're in menopausal years, it may not be a "hot flash." Some or all of the reason for body heat could stem from acute or chronic dehydration.

A very well-known and respected medical doctor and nutritionist found that 80% of all physical ills stem from lack of water. In other words, if the body were fully hydrated it would experience 80% less unpleasant physical symptoms. Isn't that astounding? 80%! Please let that sink in. 80% less physical problems!

We are continually nagged by every health professional to drink water. Most of us ignore it. I know I used to. It's annoying to have to go to the bathroom every 20-30 minutes. Eventually though, when the body starts to get the water it needs, the bladder expands, it can hold more water and the pressure to go to the bathroom as often decreases.

The tests to determine if your body is dehydrated are:

1. You feel an urgency to go to the bathroom but not much urine comes out.
2. Sometimes the urine is warm or hot.
3. Your tongue. Is it moist? If not, you're dehydrated.
4. Pull the skin on the top part of your hand between the thumb and forefinger. If it's slow to bounce back, the body is dehydrated.

If you use just one of these tests as your criteria, it may not be completely accurate. When in doubt, go with #1 and #2 as the determining tests.

Here are some other very interesting facts about water:

❧ By the time you're "thirsty," the body is already dehydrated. So, to just count on the thirst mechanism as the guide to when you should drink water is not accurate. When you're "thirsty," it's actually an alarm going off telling you that you'd better get some water in your body, fast.

❧ Skin is the largest eliminative organ. Even on days we don't sweat, the skin is releasing moisture. That moisture needs to be replaced.

❧ If a body is not getting enough water, it can get constipated easily. The bowels should eliminate three times a day. Water is the most natural laxative there is. If you're not using the bathroom three times a day, it's because the cells, tissues and organs of the body are competing for the precious liquid they have desperately needed for a long time. Eventually when you're drinking your required quota of water, the body will be hydrated enough so the three daily bowel movements will happen naturally.

❧ Oftentimes "hunger" is satisfied by drinking water which means the body wasn't hungry for food after all, but water. In 37% of Americans, the thirst mechanism is so weak that it is often mistaken for hunger.

❧ One glass of water will shut down midnight hunger pangs for almost 100% of dieters.

❧ If you're feeling stiff much of the time, it's from lack of water.

❧ Lack of water is the #1 trigger of daytime fatigue.

❧ Some preliminary research indicated that 8-10 glasses of water a day can significantly ease back and joint pain for up to 80% of sufferers.

❧ Even mild dehydration will slow down one's metabolism about 3%.

❧ A mere 2% drop in body water can trigger fuzzy short-term memory.

Sometimes even when you're drinking your quota of water, your body can still be dehydrated, especially in the summertime. Most of the reason for that is that you need more electrolytes: potassium, sodium, calcium and magnesium and trace minerals.

I have found one of the best ways of getting the body hydrated quickly is coconut water, the water inside the coconut. It has high amounts of the basic electrolytes, especially potassium. It absorbs beautifully into your system and is extremely revitalizing. Many health-food stores are selling it packaged now. It comes in plain and naturally flavored. I put the plain coconut water with frozen or fresh berries and a little of my greens powder into a blender and drink up. It's divine. You can also drink the coconut water by itself for a wonderful pick-up instead of soft drinks. Try it. You'll see.

How to determine your daily quota of water is coming up soon.

Water, Water Everywhere!

WHICH KIND DO I DRINK?

It's so easy to go round and round on that one isn't it? What I'm about to say may be met with disagreement but maybe it will make sense to you when this confusing subject is more clarified.

The best kinds of water to drink are: 1) Distilled water, 2) Spring Water that comes straight out of a natural springs and, 3) "Batch" Alkaline water.

DISTILLED WATER

Dr. Ian Shillington says it is true that distilled water will leach some minerals from the body, but the majority of these minerals are inorganic minerals you don't want anyway. Any good minerals that might possibly be leached out are more than replaced by taking minerals and trace minerals.

He also says that if inorganic minerals (and other substances like chlorine, heavy metals, bacteria, etc.) are removed from tap water by converting it into pure distilled water, the result is improved absorption of all nutrients, including minerals, and improved elimination of wastes at the cellular level. This is very important to help detoxify the body.

Is it good to use distilled water when you are making herb tea? Yes! Distilled water is empty. It has the ability to pull all the nutrients out of the herbs you put in the water.

Distilled water has been tested to be on the acidic side. Add baking soda to your water to bring it to the pH level of 7.2

If you don't have a company that delivers distilled water in glass or even if you do, a very good investment is a water distiller. Make sure you get one that uses only stainless steel parts where the water comes in contact.

SPRING WATER

It's been found that some of the "spring water" actually comes from tap water with the resultant toxins left in the water.

Most bottled mineral water purchased in stores has inorganic minerals not easily used by the body.

How do you find a good source of bottled water? We use a water company that delivers water in five-gallon glass containers to our home. Every three weeks we order a minimum of three bottles. I always feel safe drinking both their distilled and spring water. Their website is: www.mountainvalleyspring.com. When you go to their website, click on "Why Our Water is so Special" and you will see their water comes directly from a mountain spring.

To find out if there is a franchise located near you, click on "Find a Distributor" and then run your cursor over the bottles of water on the screen. A form will come up to fill in either your city or location and it will tell you if they deliver in your area. You can also order online but it's a lot more expensive as the bottles only come in liter size. I would suggest ordering just the plain water, not sparkling.

If they don't deliver in your area, find out if there's another company in your area that delivers water in glass bottles. Make sure you fully check out the quality of their water and where it comes from. A lot of the water companies, even if they don't have glass containers, have plastic ones that apparently don't affect the water. To be safe, ask the company if they've had any independent testing done to determine if their plastic leaches into the water. Make them show you the results of the testing before you drink their water.

Drinking water out of glass not only tastes much better but any concerns or doubts about water quality are eliminated.

ALKALINE WATER

Alkaline water is becoming very popular for its healing qualities. As we've covered earlier, an acid condition is one of the top reasons for hair-loss and aging. A body in an acidic condition has aches and pains and is more prone to illness and disease than a body with more of an alkaline pH.

Symptoms of an acid body are excessive falling hair, acne, agitation, dizziness, low energy, food allergies, chemical sensitivities, bloating and rapid heartbeat. These are just some of the beginning symptoms. Some of the intermediate symptoms are depression, loss of memory and concentration, migraine headaches, insomnia, ear aches, asthma, numbness and tingling. The advanced symptoms are serious illnesses.

I hope this helps you see why it's so important to get the body into the proper alkaline state.

Remember, you can add baking soda to your water which alkalizes it. Get some pH strips from a drug store and test the water. Add baking soda until it gets to 7.0 – 7.2 pH.

A "Batch" alkaline machine uses a different method than others which is far superior than other alkaline machines. The machine is worth the investment for a lifetime of health for you and your family.

It's good to alternate between distilled, spring and alkaline water. If one's system is too acidic, the alkaline water will help balance the pH. Distilled water is also important to drink because it helps detoxify the body by removing cellular waste.

When you drink water you can trust, the difference in how you feel is dramatic. I drink distilled water when I want to detoxify. I drink spring water for the natural minerals. I drink alkaline water when my pH is on the acid side.

See the Products section at www.themodernrapunzel.com for a private distributor of the Batch Alkalizer.

There's also a lot of controversy about Reverse Osmosis and Ozonated Water. I do not have the technical facts about it so I will not advise on it. If you're not sure, please do your own research.

If you're unsure, my suggestion is to try drinking several kinds of water over a long enough period of time to determine the difference in how you feel with each.

WATER CONTAMINATION

Drinking water bottled in plastic has been found to be *extremely* harmful as the toxins from the plastic can leach into the water. Bottled water shipped in trucks is prone to leaching due to the heat inside the trucks. Some plastic is heavier grade so the danger is not quite as high. But one way or another, plastic, along with polluting our bodies pollutes the environment, our waterways and oceans terribly. It's time to do away with plastic altogether. Unreal? Maybe. Vital? Yes. Do your own research. You'll be shocked at what you find. I have my strong doubts about consuming anything in plastic, no matter how "safe."

Water contamination is a big source of difficulties with hair, skin and health. There are few, if any, places in the US where the town or city water is pure. We have to drink water. We have to take showers or baths. Exposing yourself daily to these toxins is unnecessary when it can be avoided by pure water and a chlorine filter for the showers and baths. There are safe and health-giving systems for the entire house and swimming pool that completely eliminate toxins, chlorine, and chemicals.

See the Product Section at www.themodernrapunzel.com for house filtration systems.

Get chlorine filters for your shower and your sink, no matter where you live, and drink distilled, pure spring and/or alkaline water. If you don't have a filtration system in your house, wear rubber gloves when doing dishes.

Your hair and your body will love you for it. And your hair will start to gain sheen and come alive very quickly.

CHLORINE—THAT DASTARDLY CULPRIT

Science News says:

"*Chlorine is universally recognized and used as an effective chemical for purifying water. Chlorine attacks organic matter, making it a potent bleaching agent.*

"If chlorine works so well in killing bacteria and bleaching or oxidizing food stains, what does it do to our skin, eyes and lungs... all of which are organic matter! Chlorine plays havoc with our skin and hair because it chemically bonds with the protein in our bodies. It makes hair brittle and dry; it can make sensitive skin dry, flaky and itchy."

I live in a town where the water is so heavily chlorinated that you can actually smell the chlorine in a glass of water. Years ago before I started using a chlorine shower filter, my hair became so straw-like that I had to cut most of it off. Chlorine creates a chemical build-up that robs the hair of life and coats it so that it loses its sheen. During the same time I was swimming in chlorinated swimming pools. I had constant ear infections and some physical difficulties due to the chlorine my body was absorbing. Now I swim only in chlorine-free pools or the ocean and have none of those problems.

ADDITIONAL INFORMATION CONCERNING WATER CONTAMINATION

It's important to know that as much as seventy percent of municipal water systems surveyed are polluted with potentially toxic amounts of fluoride and chlorine. No matter what, it's smart to never drink right out of the tap unless you live in a completely unpolluted environment. Even then it's wise to have the water tested for contaminants before you drink it.

You're taking your life in your hands by drinking water with chlorine and toxins in it. The gases that emit from chlorine in a shower or bath are very toxic. When breathed in, chlorine damages the lungs. When chlorine is taken in through the body via drinking water, showers, baths, and swimming pools or doing dishes, it creates an environment in the body allowing for an overgrowth of harmful bacteria.

Good, clean, pure water is essential to your physical health.

HOW MUCH AND HOW OFTEN SHOULD WE CONSUME WATER?

We've been told the best way to consume water is eight ounces eight to ten times a day. But that's without taking into account the weight of the person. A woman who weighs 110 pounds is certainly not going to need the same amount of water that a man who weighs 200 pounds does.

Drinking eight ounces at a time is unproductive. The kidneys can't handle that much water at one time. Per Dr. Carey Reams, all the organs, especially the liver, do best with four ounces (six ounces in the summer due to sweating) every half hour.

Here's how you find the right amount of water for your body: Take your body weight and divide it by two. That's the amount of water in ounces to drink daily for your weight. For example, if you weigh 150 pounds, you would drink 75 ounces a day, 4 ounces at a time, every half hour. For quite a while, I used a small timer set to buzz on the half hour. Now I have a built-in "timer."

It's helpful to put your daily quota of water in glass jars first thing in the morning. Most of the time, your full quota will be consumed well before the end of the day.

When I switched to drinking four ounces of water every half hour equaling one-half my body weight every day, my energy level improved dramatically. And I look and feel *much better and much younger*!

Is there any function or organ in the body that does not benefit and heal from drinking the daily needed amount of *pure* water? The answer is: not one.

Are you drinking your quota of water for your body weight every day?

If not, let me say to you what my nutritionist said to me, over and over for months until I really got it –

Drink your quota of water every day.

Drink up my friends! Your body will love you for it and you'll notice a world of difference in your health and energy.

I promise.

Chapter Ten

Diet For Your Hair

Mother Nature Loves You

air needs nutrition to grow and replenish.
Your body is inherently strong and thrives when
you take advantage of Mother Nature's bountiful
supply of delicious whole foods. When given the proper raw materials,
the body blooms.

Put faith in Mother Nature for the healer she is. Operating otherwise
is going against natural law. Never underestimate her power. More and
more people are becoming aware of her gifts through their own personal
experience.

Going against Mother Nature is like trying to stop the sun from
shining. It's futile and unworkable.

The simple truth of having and maintaining healthy hair is a healthful
diet, one that Mother Nature has provided. Otherwise she wouldn't have
endowed planet Earth with such an abundance of marvelous foods.

Mother Nature; the only true healer for our bodies. She will reward
you with health and radiance.

THE DIVINE PLAN

Did Mother Nature include in her Divine Plan white bread, white sugar and
processed foods? No. Man has removed the life-giving nutrients from her foods.

Our vegetable gardens are not naturally laden with synthetic insecticides and pesticides. They are added. That's not part of Her Plan.

Any time food is consumed in a processed, un-whole form, *it is stored as a toxin*. And every time we consume processed food we are ignoring what was put here on Earth to keep our bodies strong, happy and healthy. It's so simple it hurts. And yet we commit the daily sin of contributing to the pollution of our bodies and this planet. It is *essential* that we provide our bodies with whole foods from Mother Nature. The health and fullness of your hair and your body depend upon it.

In 1951, Dr. Royal Lee, a true pioneer in nutrition said:

> *"One of the biggest tragedies of human civilization is the precedence of chemical therapy over nutrition. It's a substitution of artificial therapy over natural, of poisons over food, in which we are feeding people poison in trying to correct the reactions of starvation."*

Anyone who tells you directly or indirectly to ignore Mother Nature is uneducated in the truth. They aren't observing the obvious. They have bought "authority" and are ignoring the real Authority of Mother Nature.

The body requires certain fuels to function properly. When it is not given the fuel it was initially designed to utilize, it has to readjust, taking energy away from various organs, muscles and tissues to compensate. Then it becomes overwhelmed or rebels. Toxic build-up occurs as the eliminative organs: kidneys, liver, intestines and skin, become exhausted and can't do their job. The body can barely keep up, if at all, with the input of foods it was not designed to handle.

Jonny Bowden, PhD, Certified Nutritionist and author of several best-selling books on health says:

> *"Eat real food. Food your grandmother would have recognized as food. Food you could hunt, fish, gather or pluck. Food as close to its natural form as possible. Food without a bar code. Whole fruit (not the fruit juice). Whole eggs (not the egg whites). Meat, eggs and milk from healthy, grass-fed*

cows and chickens that roam around pecking at worms (free-range). Any vegetable in the world."

Your body has the ability to replenish itself twenty-four hours a day when given the right building blocks. Just as you wouldn't put dirt in your gas tank because it wouldn't run well if you did, the body operates on certain clear-cut laws — that of Mother Nature.

Respect her. Honor her. Listen to her. Heed her messages. She's trying to make you whole. She speaks the truth. You don't need to look for her. She's already here.

Let her help you achieve the health and head of hair you deserve.

Are You Confused About What to Eat?

Welcome to the club!

The Standard American Diet is "S.A.D." More and more people are becoming aware of the fact that what we eat affects how we look and how we feel. But the many questions about diet still remain.

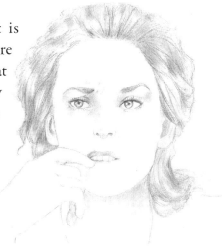

Have you noticed that just about every book, every person you talk to says something different about what's good for you and what's not good for you to eat? There's hardly any food item on the planet that one "authority" says to eat and another says not to! Have you ever felt your limited and restrained options for what you can and should eat has left you hanging by a carrot and not even sure you should eat that?

Remember the movie "Network" when Peter Finch yells out the window to everyone within earshot, "I'm mad as hell and I'm not going to take it anymore!" I don't know about you, but that's how I used to feel.

"You should drink milk" versus "Don't drink milk; milk is only for babies." "Eat meat" versus "Don't eat anything with a face." "Wheat is bad for you." "Don't eat any veggies that grow below ground." Haven't heard that one? Yes, some have that opinion. "Don't eat eggs." "Don't eat cheese," etc, etc, etc. All the "don'ts" leave only the question of "What are the "*dos*"?

So what's the real story? Were or are our grandparents so wrong when they said to eat a balanced diet made up of wholesome foods? (Note the "*whole*" in "wholesome," as in *whole* grains.) Did they not have and use just good, ole' common sense?

As a child I had no clue about healthy foods. A lot of times for breakfast I was fed white bread with powdered sugar and concentrated orange juice. I remember spending the night at my Grandmothers and the next morning she gave me whole-wheat toast and fresh orange juice. I thought I was being poisoned! I was so upset I called my Mom and asked her to please come get me. Little did I know!

Here's a simple guideline to help sort through the multitude of confusions. I hope it helps *a lot*.

The Rules:

1. If it sounds good and it's good for you, eat it.
2. If it doesn't sound good even if it's healthy, don't eat it.
3. If it's unhealthy and sounds good, don't eat it.

That's one "do" and two "don'ts." If all you remember is #1, you'll do great as long as you stick to it on the long-term.

Our desire for different kinds of foods changes all the time. That's a good thing. *We need variety*. Follow your instincts when you're standing over the fruit and vegetable section in your grocery store or farmer's market. If you feel you "should" eat those parsnips, even though they sound disgusting, do not touch them. They won't be good for you. Grab those items that sound and look good and are good for you. If eating bell peppers sounds like a dream come true, go for it! Whatever is in those bell peppers, your body is telling you it needs.

Once in a while I get a craving for a steak. And boy do I enjoy that steak. But if I ate that steak because I felt I "should," it wouldn't go down my throat happily no matter how many enzymes I took to digest it.

Did you see the movie "Annie Hall" with Woody Allen? Woody Allen was not your health-food kinda guy. If you remember the scene in the health-food restaurant in Los Angeles when he ordered "smashed beans with sprouts," you'll appreciate someone trying to stomach something just because it's "healthy." I laughed 'til I cried. He was trying to figure out how to "get in the groove" and impress Annie. It didn't work.

WEIGHT—HOW AM I GOING TO LOSE IT AND KEEP IT OFF?

When foods are consumed that the body does not recognize as nutrition (processed foods), it stores them. And guess what? Overweight problems can stem from stored, undigested food.

It's been said that Americans are overfed but under-nourished. When the body is not getting what it needs, it's constantly hungry–not for more bulk but for nutrition. When whole nutrient-dense foods are eaten in smaller quantities, the body is not begging for more and more food as it's getting what it needs.

Most of the weight problem in America is not what most people think it is. It is simply that the body is not getting what it needs and it keeps saying, "Feed me, feed me what I need!" Instead it's loaded down with "food" the body doesn't recognize, foods not in their original state, food that is now stored as weight.

If emphasis was on long-term correct nutrition, it would make sense that a lot of weight problems would resolve. The power of the body to rejuvenate and balance itself is amazing. But we all want the "quick fix." That's become the American way. Crash diets will only put weight right back on when the diet is over as the problem still exists–lack of the proper nutrients.

Losing and then maintaining proper weight requires eating small, highly-nutritious meals as often as needed to keep one's blood-sugar balanced. Smaller and more frequent nutrient-dense meals a day can sustain energy and won't overload the body with too much food at one time.

Have you ever noticed how your body gets sluggish (if not exhausted) after a big meal? It's just too big a load on the entire digestive system. Too much food at one time makes digestion difficult, especially at night.

If you're trying to lose weight, work on eliminating dairy, beef (except very lean meats) and fried foods. These are high-fat foods. Walk 35–40 minutes a day. This will increase your fat-burning ability and improve digestion. Eat veggies and high-quality protein. That combination sheds weight.

Don't try to lose weight too quickly. One to two pounds a week is ideal. Weight will stay off when it comes off gradually.

Whole, nutrient-dense foods, in their unbroken state, can always be relied upon to give you health and long life. Before you know it, the pounds start coming off because you're getting real nutrition instead of deficient, empty food that only puts on unhealthy pounds.

Compare the difference between fruit and vegetables; vibrant and alive, versus processed food; dull and lifeless.

Need I say more?

BACK TO BASICS AGAIN

Remember when we used to hear about "a balanced diet"? Each meal needs to include small amounts of food that: a) will give you instant energy like leafy vegetables, b) whole grains or starchy vegetables and c) protein that sounds good to you. If you've wanted to go on a vegetarian diet and have been concerned you won't get enough protein, here are some interesting facts. There are 7 grams of protein per ounce in steak. There are 13 grams of protein in one cup of dry beans. There are 4 grams of protein in one cup of broccoli. Most of us don't know that vegetables and beans contain high-quality protein. And you can't beat the other benefits they provide in terms of vitamins and minerals.

All three will sustain you and give you the energy you need until your next meal.

I used to think I could and should eat only fruit and vegetables because most everything else will lead to a disaster of some kind. We're led to believe that. It's just not true.

I'm sure you've already heard that you need to eat a nutritious breakfast, a little larger meal at lunch and the smallest at dinner so you're not going to bed with a full stomach. It's true. The body needs to rejuvenate at night, not digest. If you need to snack in-between meals, here's a suggestion. Have a small handful of your favorite raw nuts with a piece of fruit or some celery with your favorite nut butter. Stay away from anything with sugar or corn syrup in it. Sugar will spike your blood-sugar and then crash, making you tired. Have small "snacks" that are delicious and healthy.

TEST YOURSELF

The easiest way to know if something is good for your body is to eat it and see how you feel afterwards. It's good if you didn't get a stomach-ache but it's great if you derive energy out of the food which is what food is supposed to do–give you energy, enough energy to last until your next meal which sugar and processed items will never do!

If the food item you just ate robbed you of energy, even if it's healthy, eliminate it for awhile. You may be getting too much of that one food too often. It's best not to eat the same food three days in a row. By doing that, we help avoid food allergies. Our bodies thrive with variety.

ON-GOING DIET REGIMEN

- Eat a balanced diet of organic fruits, vegetables, grains and protein. Whenever possible, choose local organic food.
- Eat fruits and vegetables that sound good to you and are in season. *For ideal health*, 80% of your diet should be organic fruits and vegetables. If you eat this way and drink fresh fruit and vegetable juices daily, you'll find your need for supplements is greatly reduced or perhaps eventually not needed at all.
- It's best to eat half of your vegetables raw and the other half cooked. For cooked vegetables, steam or bake them but do not boil them unless you drink the cooking water. When vegetables are boiled, the nutrients end up in the water, not in your body. A salad with a variety of raw vegetables for lunch and lightly steamed vegetables for dinner provides you with essential fiber, vitamins and minerals. Some people have trouble digesting raw

Garden Produce

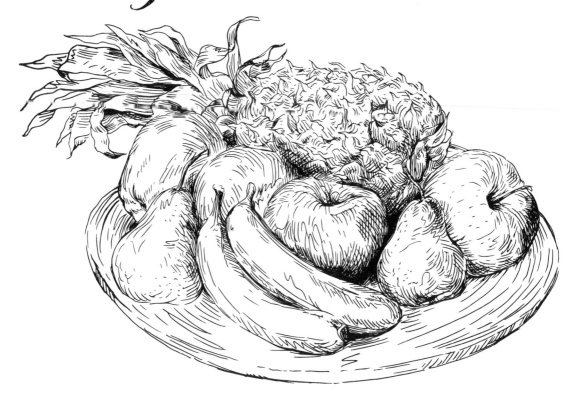

Love Fruits

vegetables. In that case, eat all steamed vegetables until you're able to digest the raw vegetables too.

❧ Sauté only with sesame, olive or coconut oil at low temperatures.

❧ Consume meats that are hormone and antibiotic-free. It's ideal to find beef that is grass-fed and fish that is caught from rivers or oceans, not farm-raised.

❧ Raw, unpasteurized dairy products. Some people do great on them, others not. Contact a local dairy farmer that sells them.

❧ Eat small to medium size portions of nutrient-dense, balanced meals three times a day. Smaller portions put much less strain on the digestive system. You should only eat until your stomach is three-quarters full. One of the best books I've found for nutrient-dense recipes is by Dr. Joel Fuhrman. You can find it on Amazon books. It's called: *Eat for Health: Lose Weight, Keep It Off, Look Younger, Live Longer* (2 Volume Set).

❧ Chew your food slowly and thoroughly while savoring the taste. The saliva in your mouth is a natural enzyme that helps digest food. Raw foods have their own enzymes, especially papaya and pineapple. You can eat these two delicious fruits with any meal to help with digestion.

❧ Do not drink liquids with meals at all or very little. Drinking fluids with meals washes away the natural digestive juices your body produces. Drink only that amount needed to swallow supplements.

❧ Whole grains provide B vitamins for energy, fiber and complete carbohydrates for fuel. If you have digestive problems, avoid wheat, rye, barley and corn and eat brown rice, buckwheat, oatmeal and millet instead. It's also beneficial to soak your grains overnight in pure water before you cook them the next day. This makes them easier to digest.

❧ Keep informed on the foods that are genetically modified. Stay away from them at all costs. Currently soy, corn, cottonseed oil and canola oil head the top of the list of genetically modified foods. Keep up to date with any others.

- Rotate your foods. In other words, don't eat the same thing every day. It's best not to have the same food within three days. Have a large variety of fruits and vegetables, especially the leafy greens.

- Fruit *juice* can cause bacteria and yeast overgrowth in the intestines. Eat *fresh* fruit instead. Fresh fruit and freshly made fruit juices have an abundance of anti-oxidants and healing properties found nowhere else, especially blueberries and strawberries. You can make delicious fresh fruit drinks in your blender. Add raw nuts or seeds (almonds, cashews, etc.) and one or more of coconut, oat, non-GMO soy, hemp or almond milk for a complete, balanced meal.

- Blackstrap Molasses is an amazing source of minerals and natural iron. Add it to cereals, casseroles and grains. Dark leafy vegetables and broccoli are also great sources of minerals.

- Take essential fatty acids. Excellent sources of EFA's are in avocado, nuts and seeds. Avocados contain high-quality essential fatty acids. Avocados are also a great source of minerals which support a healthy alkaline blood balance and are high in vitamin E which slows down aging. Another good omega 3, 6, 9 blend consists of 2 tablespoons of organic unrefined whole flaxseeds, 1 tablespoon of organic whole pumpkin seeds and 1 tablespoon of whole organic sunflower seeds. Blend all three until it's a powder and then add to any of your fruit or vegetable drinks. You can also sprinkle it on your salad or take 2 tablespoons straight from the spoon per day.

- Eat your dinner meal as early as possible and make it your smallest meal. Going to sleep on a full stomach can put on weight and inhibit a good night's sleep as the body is trying to digest, not rest. If you're hungry before bed, try drinking some water or have a few sips of vegetarian protein drink.

- Remember your fresh vegetable and fruit juices!

Remember health food shouldn't taste like "cardboard." Something's wrong if it does. It has to be prepared correctly. It should taste delicious to you.

As a reward for being good with your diet, go ahead and eat something you "shouldn't" once in awhile. It's okay to disagree. You're showing your body who's boss.

Rabbi Moshe Ben Maimon, born in Spain in 1135 said:

> *"Listen to one's body to achieve maximum health. As a rule, one should avoid going to extremes, but rather, each person should pursue the "middle way." One should not eat until one's stomach is completely full, but rather, should only eat until one's stomach is three-quarters full.   Overeating is like poison to the body, and is the cause of many illnesses. Most illnesses are caused by "bad foods" and by overeating respectively. (One can even overeat on good foods.)"*

He adds that warming the body stimulates the metabolism and readies the stomach for eating and digestion. Also stressed is the importance of eating foods that are easy to digest, commenting that a wise person eats a meal with very few ingredients, preferably all cooked together.

He also says, "No disease that can be treated by diet should be treated with any other means."

I hope you've found something in this section that has not only brought you some relief from the seemingly never-ending confusion of what and how to feed your body but that you can see a way to judge these things for yourself. The only way you'll know is to try out these basic concepts.

Remember; beautiful, thick hair and healthy skin starts with nutrition. Once again, here are the rules:

1. If it sounds good and it's good for you, eat it.
2. If it doesn't sound good even if it's healthy, don't eat it.
3. If it's unhealthy and sounds good, don't eat it.

For Your Hair's Sake
How to Free Yourself of Food Cravings

Here is the story of how junk-food became a thing of the past for me. I hope you find it interesting reading and very useful.

In the early 70's I decided to completely eliminate the last of my junk-food cravings. I had been strict with eating mostly healthy food for a long time.

I decided to experiment.

Every night a friend and I went to a well-known chain restaurant and I ate just what I craved: French fries, an American grilled-cheese sandwich and a hot fudge sundae.

Instead of making myself feel guilty, I decided to *thoroughly enjoy* the process. I called it "pigging-out with reverence." I relished every bite, the taste on my palette and was in awe of every morsel. No exaggeration.

I feasted on those three items for a month. At the end of the month I no longer craved the sandwiches or the chocolate shakes. I was over it. I've had none since because it doesn't sound good to me. (I must admit I still love French fries and will splurge once in a while.)

The interesting thing was how I looked. Before starting the process I didn't think I was going to look terrible when it was over. But after that month, let me tell you, I looked awful. My skin was pasty and pale, my face puffy and lumpy, my eyes looked dull and lifeless and my hair had lost its sheen and was wimpy. I looked completely different.

It was a real awakening that what I had been doing before that time had made all the difference in how I looked. It took just one month to go from looking healthy to looking at least ten years older. But I was off junk food for good. I had no more cravings.

I was done with the cravings because not only did I *not make myself guilty* for eating the fries, the shake, the sundae, I *thoroughly enjoyed them*.

How many times have you personally experienced or watched someone you know, while eating something they "shouldn't," not only not enjoy what they're eating but have "guilt" written all over their face? That alone will make it so they just have to keep doing it and keep the vicious cycle of "being bad" persisting!

Enjoy it completely, with your whole heart and soul, until you're done. You may say "What if I still crave butterscotch after a year of 'pigging out with reverence'?" It's either you didn't truly enjoy it while you were eating it or it's time to find a substitute! There are delicious substitutes without the white sugar and other toxic substances.

If processed food made one's body look and feel great, I would be in support of them and I'm sure a lot of other people would too. But those foods don't provide vitality and beauty.

One should be able to eat junk food once in awhile and have little to no bad effects. Some young people are able to get away with it for a short while but unfortunately, over time, deficiencies caused by foods without nutrition catches up. It will then show in the texture, fullness and beauty of one's hair and skin.

Be very alert to when certain foods change the way you look and feel. To stay in control, keep a detailed diary to monitor your diet and what foods affect you, good and bad. You will then know what foods to eliminate, even for a short while, and what foods are nourishing as they give you energy.

Remember the rules: If you're craving something and it's healthy, eat it. If you're craving something and it's not healthy, don't eat it. Find a healthy substitute for that unhealthy food or drink you're craving. There are many natural and tasty substitutes for colas, candy bars and processed foods.

A sugar craving can mean low blood sugar and/or a deficiency in B vitamins. Oftentimes sugar cravings diminish by eating high-quality proteins. High-quality proteins stabilize blood sugar.

If you're craving a particular fruit or vegetable, eat as much as you want for awhile. The body is telling you it needs it. If you're craving junk food, that's a different story. It's like a drug. It's addicting.

It's important your eating habits aren't changed too quickly. If one doesn't get off processed food gradually the body will detoxify too quickly. Eliminate one unhealthy item at a time (like sugar) and when you no longer crave it, eliminate another (like fried foods). Eventually you'll have little to no desire for processed food. Your taste buds will change and you'll find junk food (as in white sugar and soft drinks) that once sounded "irresistible" now sounds boring or disgusting. Your body will want only life-giving, natural, whole foods. That's a great sign you're on your way to true health and in harmony with natural law. *And it will show in the quality of your hair and skin.*

Every person I've talked to who made the decision to eat whole foods and followed through with it, has experienced the same thing; they completely lost interest in junk food and regained their health, beauty and vitality.

Hippocrates, the founding father of medicine said, *"Let food be thy medicine."*

Big No-Nos!

Listed here are some toxic substances commonly consumed. They bring the vitality of the body down to a point where the system has a very difficult time regenerating no matter how healthy one is eating.

SUGAR: THE UNIVERSAL POISON

The biggest "no-no" is sugar, which is why a full page is dedicated to it.

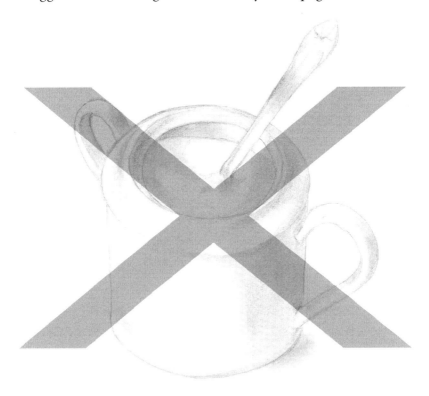

Refined sugar is the number one toxic product pushed by food industries throughout every nation. Dr. Ian Shillington says that beyond any doubt whatsoever, products that have refined sugar in them create disastrous consequences. He goes on to say that sugar is the primary physical cause of Diabetes, Fatigue, Obesity, Impotence, Colds, Flu, Fibromyalgia, Immune system disorders, Liver and Kidney problems and a thousand other harmful conditions. When you add more processed food to the equation, you have the complete picture of a dangerous, life-threatening situation.

He goes on to say that the apparency of these so-called "foods" provides energy, and yet this "boost" is very short-lived and very destructive of the body. There is absolutely no nutritional value to sugar, only damage. White sugar is not a whole food; the essential health-giving element, molasses, has been removed.

Nutritious white sugar substitutes are: honey, real maple syrup (not synthetic), agave, date sugar, molasses, brown rice syrup, stevia and barley malt. The darker the sweetener, the more minerals it has.

White sugar depletes B vitamins, the anti-stress vitamin. B vitamins are *essential* for hair growth and make stress much easier to cope with.

I once saw a film of children who were diagnosed with psychiatric disorders. The real cause of the "disorder" was due to food allergies. This was proven through ceasing the use of the offending food allergen and then no longer having the "mental" symptom. It was absolutely *amazing* to watch. It was like night and day. Sugar = completely insane! No sugar = normal. There were also, individually for each child, other foods causing similar allergic reactions. You'd never believe it unless you watched it yourself. It was dramatic.

How many psychotropic drugs are being prescribed when the real cause of "mental problems" stem from food allergies or environmental sensitivities (as in toxic household substances)? Proper diagnosis is *essential*. When the correct problem is found it is solved.

BARBEQUED FOODS

These foods are known to be carcinogenic so it's best to avoid them completely, especially those with digestive problems.

FRIED FOODS

Foods fried in anything but sesame, olive or coconut oil at low temperature are very difficult to digest. They make the skin break out, cause it to be puffy and blotchy and the scalp congested. Potato chips, French fries and fried chicken are some examples. Stay away from them.

COCA-COLA

To carry the Coca-Cola syrup concentrate, the commercial trucks must display a hazardous-material sign. The distributors of Coke have been using it to clean the engines in their trucks for about 20 years. Coke will dissolve a nail in four days.

Coke leaches calcium from bone and is a major contributor to the rise in osteoporosis.

"Useful" purposes:

To clean a toilet, pour a can of Coca-Cola into the toilet bowl and let it sit for one hour, then flush clean. To remove rust spots from chrome car bumpers, rub the bumper with a rumpled-up piece of Reynolds Wrap aluminum foil dipped in Coca-Cola. To clean corrosion from car battery terminals, pour a can of Coca-cola over the terminals to bubble away the corrosion. To loosen a rusted bolt, apply a cloth soaked in Coca-cola to the rusted bolt for several minutes.

Now the question is, would you like a glass of water for your body instead? Keep a bottle of Coke around for the above "useful" purposes, which don't include consuming it.

CAFFEINE

A friend of mine, Kathy Rose Willis, has done extensive research and found the following information about caffeine.

Here is some, but far from all, of the research she has done:

People use caffeine because they think it gives them energy. In truth, caffeine produces fake energy in your body and, in the process, causes all kinds of problems.

» *Caffeine dehydrates your body, which can cause headaches, muscle aches and degeneration of organs as well as wrinkles.*

- *It causes the loss of potassium, zinc, magnesium, vitamins B & C and reduces the absorption of iron and calcium from foods which can lead to osteoporosis, anemia, and hormonal imbalances with resulting aggravated PMS and menopausal symptoms, including hot flashes, panic, anxiety and mood swings.*
- *It stimulates your adrenals, eventually overworking those glands and leading to adrenal exhaustion which can cause fatigue, a weakened immune system, impaired digestion, sexual dysfunction, anxiety and panic attacks.*
- *It makes your body more acid, increasing the risk of degenerative diseases, especially cancer.*
- *It increases your heart rate and blood pressure and ages your body faster.*
- *It decreases the quality of your sleep, thereby contributing to morning grogginess and the need for more artificial stimulants and/or sleeping pills.*
- *It interferes with carbohydrate metabolism and proper liver function, contributing to obesity and weight-loss problems.*

Most coffee is loaded with pesticides which cause their own health problems. There is not one good thing that it does besides making you feel high temporarily. Caffeine is not a nutrient needed by the body to survive! Instead it is a highly addictive drug, needing larger and larger amounts for an effect and causing painful withdrawal when you quit using it suddenly.

If all the effects of coffee as listed above were on the label on every coffee cup in the country, how many less cups would be sold daily? People just don't know that a majority of their health problems are connected with this highly addictive "beverage" they drink several times a day.

Don't take my word for it, but read what clinical nutritionist, Stephen Cherniske, M.S. has to say in his book, Caffeine Blues, regarding how it affects every system in your body. If you really want a beautiful body you need to take a look at this. Do you value your life and your health enough to want to make the change?

Caffeine comes from many sources and is present in many products. Most people think of coffee and black tea when they hear that word, but it is also in white tea and green tea to a lesser degree, yerba mate tea, colas, hot chocolate and chocolate candies, and is in many energy drinks from a source

*called guarana. Many over-the-counter drugs, some bottled waters and even
"health" products have it added so you have to read the labels.*

THE REMEDY

Kathy goes on to say:

*Because of the addictive nature of caffeine and the fact that the body is thrown
so out of whack by it, quitting needs to be done gradually, not cold-turkey,
unless you want a whopper headache and possibly extreme fatigue and depression for a couple days.*

*The first thing to do to quit caffeine is to make a decision to join the group of
people who want to be healthier. Then get a good green drink to help alkalize
your body. The first day drink it once, then twice the next day, then three
times daily for about a week. You should notice that the more you do this,
the less coffee you will want and need. After that week start decreasing your
caffeine intake by watering down what you are drinking or just using less
every day until you feel you can do without it.*

*Meanwhile, keep drinking your green drink two or three times a day. Just
keep at it until you can say you are caffeine-free and then continue to use
highly nutritious foods and products, particularly green drinks, whole food
supplements and raw juices to give your body more life and real energy so it
doesn't need the fake energy from caffeine anymore.*

MSG- MONOSODIUM GLUTAMATE

John Erb, author of *The Slow Poisoning of America*, made an amazing
discovery while going through scientific journals in his research on MSG.
He wondered if there could be an actual chemical causing the massive
obesity epidemic.

He found that MSG triples the amount of insulin the pancreas creates;
causing rats (and humans?) to become obese.

He says that MSG is added to food for the addictive effect it has on the
human body and that food producers and restaurants have been addicting
us to their products for years and now we are paying the price. MSG is
in the foods in our favorite coffee shops, drive-ups and packaged food
commonly consumed.

MSG hides behind names such as Natural Flavoring, Hydrolyzed Vegetable Protein, Accent and Natural Meat Tenderizer. It's shocking to see just how many of the foods consumed every day have this poison in them, especially the "healthy low-fat" foods.

This gives just one more great reason to listen to Mother Nature and avail ourselves of the whole, unprocessed, additive-free foods she provides!

Try to eat at home whenever possible. If you buy canned food, look at the labels before you buy them.

MICROWAVE OVENS

As we know, a microwave oven cooks food at very high temperatures. When food is cooked at high temperatures, vital nutrients are destroyed. Food should be cooked at low temperatures for longer periods of time to preserve the nutrients.

A slow-cooker is a very good way to go. It not only preserves those vital nutrients but the food tastes better because it's wholesome.

We are the recipients of radiation from electronics. Why unnecessarily radiate our foods? A good example of what happens with food that is *not* radiated is a potato which has its little buds on it. Over time those buds will start to sprout which means it's alive; whereas if that potato was radiated it will not sprout. Unfortunately not all foods give us that obvious indicator which is why it's important to avoid radiating foods altogether.

ASPARTAME

Do you know anyone who drinks diet soda or chews sugar-free gum? Here is some information for you from Dr. Joseph Mercola:

> *"Aspartame is a poison that does not belong in your body and this is not an exaggeration. Yet, this toxic substance is consumed by over 200 million people around the world and is found in more than 6,000 products. Everything from soda and chewing gum to desserts, yogurt, and even some vitamins and cough drops contain it. When you drink, say, a can of diet soda sweetened with aspartame, what are you really consuming?"*

To see how aspartame damages the brain, I suggest doing your own Internet research on it. It's scary.

These "Big No-Nos" have been added to this book because they are, each one, a major drain on the energy of the body. When they are eliminated, one's physical well-being isn't being continually sabotaged while trying to implement and benefit from the procedures in this book.

Why consume these poisonous substances when later they will only need to be detoxified from your body? Make it easier on yourself. Eliminate them.

To end off this chapter let me share a parable a friend sent me:

"In the beginning, God created the Heavens and the Earth and populated the Earth with green, yellow and red vegetables of all kinds so Man and Woman would live long and healthy lives.

"Then Satan created Ice Cream and Donuts. And Satan said, 'You want chocolate with that?' And Man said, 'Yes!' and Woman said, 'and as long as you're at it, add some sprinkles.' And they gained 10 pounds. And Satan smiled.

"And God created the healthful yogurt that Woman might keep the figure that Man found so fair. And Satan brought forth white flour from the wheat and white sugar from the cane and combined them. And Woman went from size 6 to size 16.

"So God said, 'Try my fresh green salad.' And Satan presented Thousand-Island Dressing, buttery croutons and garlic toast on the side. And Man and Woman unfastened their belts.

"God then said, 'I have sent you heart-healthy vegetables and olive oil in which to cook them.' And Satan brought forth deep-fried fish and chicken-fried steak. And Man and Woman gained more weight and their cholesterol went through the roof.

"Satan then created chocolate cake and named it 'Devil's Food.'

"Then God brought forth the potato, naturally low in fat and brimming with nutrition. And Satan peeled off the healthful skin and sliced the starchy center into chips and deep-fried them. And Man and Woman gained pounds.

"God then gave Man lean beef so that Man might consume fewer calories and still satisfy his appetite. And Satan created 99-cent double cheeseburgers. Then said, 'You want fries with that?' And Man replied, 'Yes! And super size them!' And Satan said, 'It is good.'

"God then brought forth running shoes so that His children might lose those extra pounds. And Satan gave cable TV with a remote control so Man would not have to toil changing the channels. And Man and Woman watched the flickering light and gained pounds."

Enough said.

Chapter Eleven

Vitamins, Chiropractic and Exercise—Do They Really Make a Difference?

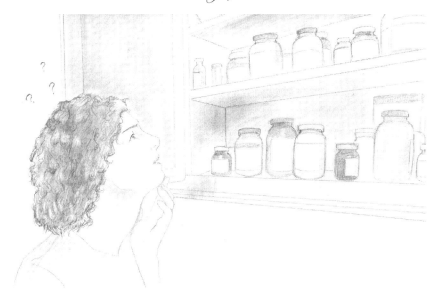

Vitamins

There is a great deal of confusion and controversy about vitamins and supplements, just like there is diet.

First of all, why is it important to take vitamins for our health and beauty? The answer is because they are "supplements." Let me explain. Vitamins and minerals supplement what we're not getting from food due to poor soil and processed foods. Women had long beautiful hair in other times because they were getting the nutrients they needed from food grown in nutrient-rich soil. They didn't need supplements.

If we ate fruit and vegetables grown in rich organic soil, it's doubtful we would need supplements. The exception is when one is experiencing undue stress which requires additional nutritional support.

If you don't have your own garden and orchard or access to an abundance of organic food grown in nutrient-rich soil, you may ask these questions: "What vitamins do I take?" "How do I know they'll work and make me feel better like they're supposed to before I invest my hard-earned money in them?" It's easy to hesitate buying vitamins at all by not knowing the answers to these valid questions.

If you've done research on your own or have talked with friends who are taking good care of themselves, you've probably discovered that there are an enormous number of supplements on the market designed to handle this or that symptom. And more continue to be developed to keep up with the needs of modern times.

If you've taken up the challenge of trying to find which one will help a troublesome symptom and have ended up over time with one or more cupboards packed to overflowing with unused supplements (representing hundreds perhaps even thousands of dollars), then it's possible you may be disillusioned enough not to bother with supplements at all, or very little. One is then forced to go seek another solution that may not be wise; a solution that will only cause more serious problems over time.

The quote by C. W. Ceran, *"Genius is the ability to reduce the complicated to the simple"* is the real trick to living. But it shouldn't be a trick at all. Simple is truth. Complicated is, well... complicated.

Let's get simple. The body has certain basic needs. Now before you possibly object to what I'm about to say, just bear with me and see if what is said here makes sense to you. Let me cite the time I spoke to a brilliant doctor about a confusion so many people face.

"CLINICAL NUTRITION"

A few years ago, I was teaching in Montana. A friend of mine told me about a chiropractor there in case I needed one. I went to see him and learned something that made complete sense.

"Clinical nutrition" has become a fad. That's where the doctor or nutritionist gives the patient one or more isolated nutrients to handle deficiencies or handle a particular symptom. We know vitamin and mineral deficiencies are vital to handle. But this doctor, who has been in practice for over forty years, discovered something very interesting in dealing with the chronic problems his patients were facing with their health. He found that the patients who were *continually* using isolated supplements to handle this or that symptom eventually became worse and worse.

The reason for that is those supplements that were given, were given without attention to *balance*, and many times they were creating other deficiencies. In this case, the body can, over time, become extremely confused.

I witnessed this in a family member of mine. Her "clinical nutrition" became the habit of taking handfuls of supplements at a time to handle her symptoms. Her condition worsened and continued to do so. After all the hard work, years and cost she put in to trying to get well, she got to the point of apathy. Needless to say, it was *very* upsetting.

This doctor, upon seeing the same "result" in some of his patients, those who had long-term chronic physical problems, told them he was not going to give them any more isolated supplements. He only gave them the standard live vitamins the body needs on a regular basis: Vitamin A, Vitamin B, Vitamin C, Vitamin D, Vitamin E and all the minerals, in the right balance. It took some of the patients two to three months for their bodies to adapt and some went through a tough time while their bodies were becoming balanced, but they all healed.

Too many people become frantic if something doesn't work right away. The "feel better quick" has become a drug in its own way. "If it doesn't work *now*, then forget it!" That's a choice everyone has to make. It can take some time.

Many times one *does* needs to take other supplements along with the basics. For example, if one lives in a polluted area, it's essential to take anti-oxidants. Taking a supplement to solve a deficiency on a temporary basis is many times required for health. The point is not to get immersed in supplements your body doesn't have a clue how to deal with. To make "clinical nutrition" the overall solution ignores the basic requirements of the body on a long-term basis.

Start with the basics always. The body requires these. See your nutritionist to determine what other supplements you may need along with the basics, if any.

VITAMINS AND MINERALS

In this day and age most of the fruits and vegetables are grown in soil deficient of vitamins and minerals. It didn't used to be that way. Unfortunately most of us have to supplement. Some of the symptoms caused by lack of the basic vitamins are:

Vitamin A: acne, wrinkles, aging skin, dry hair, peeling nails, night blindness, impaired vision and many others.

Vitamin B: hair loss, acne, eczema, yellow skin, oily skin, whiteheads, pale skin, stretch marks, sore mouth, exhaustion, burning pains, tiredness, inflammation of the lips, lack of concentration, depression, lack of strength and many others.

Vitamin B12: loss of appetite, pale skin, problems concentrating, shortness of breath, diarrhea, constipation, mental confusion, depression, loss of balance and several others.

Vitamin C: acne, eczema, wrinkles, aging skin, peeling nails, bleeding under the skin, bruising, loose teeth, bleeding gums, sore arms and muscles, arthritis, difficulty in healing, fragile and brittle bones, colds, flu, infection and healing resistance, lack of endurance, wounds that won't heal, and shortness of breath.

Vitamin D: bowleggedness, retarded growth, convulsions, lack of vigor, restlessness.

Vitamin E: acne, stretch marks, wrinkles, aging skin, exhaustion, general weakness, muscle weakness.

Now you can see some of the negative effects basic vitamin deficiencies can cause. The B vitamins are especially important. Vitamin B6 is important for supporting many normal healthy body functions, including hair growth. Biotin, also a B vitamin, plays a very important role in supporting healthy skin, hair and nails.

Take the complete B complex to ensure your B vitamins are balanced and ensure that when you take B vitamins you also take the other necessary vitamins and minerals in balance. See your natural health-care professional.

LIFE IN VITAMINS

We take vitamins to feel better and have more energy. But what most people are not aware of is that the only factor that makes vitamins work is how much life they have in them. One must take into consideration how long the vitamin has been sitting on the shelf, either your shelf or the store's shelves. Taking them before the expiration date ensures optimum potency. You can take vitamins and minerals after the expiration date, but they won't be quite as potent.

SYNTHETIC VITAMINS

Most "enriched" foods such as some cereals and bread are "enriched" with synthetic (man-made) vitamins.

Vitamins must be from whole foods from Mother Nature to support health. When the body doesn't recognize them as food, it has no other alternative but to store (not assimilate) the "vitamin" as a toxin, which results in pain and poor health. Synthetic vitamins are not food, but chemicals. You might as well throw them down the drain. They're toxic.

A friend of mine recently bought chewable vitamin C tablets and found them sweetened with aspartame which is dangerous to the body. Ensure you look for additives in supplements before you buy them.

Many people believe that the nutrition industry and the pharmaceutical industry are separate powers. What many people don't know is that most of the vitamins you buy from your family-owned or chain nutrition store come from the same corporations.

Natural healing occurs only as a result of taking pure, unadulterated foods, plants, herbs, and other sea-plant nutritional sources.

When you buy vitamins, whether they're from a health-food store, online or a drug store, look at the ingredients first. Make sure they're derived from live sources. Live sources come from the actual food, not synthetically made in a laboratory.

Make sense? I hope so.

ASSIMILATION OF VITAMINS

Several years ago, an article written by the sanitation department in a major city stated that up to 80% of the sewage was undigested vitamins! Can you imagine that! Certain kinds of vitamins don't break down which makes them indigestible. You can always count on the chewables, capsules and liquids to assimilate.

If you take tablets chew them or break them up in your mouth first before swallowing. If you find you're not getting the benefit you expect from vitamins in capsules, open them up and add them to a protein drink, which makes them palatable. There's no point in wasting your hard-earned money.

One can take vitamins but until you give the body a fresh start by detoxification, they're not quite as effective. By implementing the whole process simultaneously—eating healthy, taking the right supplements and detoxification—you will make great headway. Consult your natural-health doctor for the program best for your body.

To re-cap, if you're not experiencing a noticeable difference from taking your vitamins, it's because:
  a. They're not balanced. See your nutritionist.
  b. They're not alive. Take live vitamins.
  c. They're synthetic. Take live vitamins made from real food.
  d. You're not assimilating them. Take liquid vitamins and minerals, capsules or chewables.

MINERALS

A deficiency in minerals is equally responsible for a number of hair and skin problems. For example:

Hair loss: deficiency in iron, selenium, zinc and sulfur
Hair that is coarse and brittle: deficiency in zinc
Dandruff: deficiency in magnesium
Acne: deficiency in zinc
Rashes: deficiency in calcium

There are many, many more symptoms associated with mineral deficiencies than those listed above. When you keep your body supplied with an abundance of the basic minerals and trace minerals through juicing, a healthy diet and correct supplementation, you'll get what you need for optimum health. You'll feel the difference.

It's important to note that magnesium works with calcium to promote healthy hair growth. Magnesium is the fourth most abundant mineral in the body and is *essential* to good health. Food sources of magnesium include green vegetables, wheat germ, whole grains, nuts, chickpeas and fish.

SWEATING AND LOSS OF MINERALS

Here's an interesting article written by Dr. Cindy Clayton.

Your body is a dynamic entity—this means it's characterized by constant change and activity. As a living organism, it responds to changes in the environment. Summer, with its heat and higher level of physical activity, is an environmental change you can prepare for.

Summer puts specific stresses on your body and your health.

If your adrenals are weak, your body can't balance salt and potassium. Correct balance of these two minerals is necessary for good health and simply feeling good. Your body's ability to sweat adequately-but not excessively-for the purpose of cooling and detoxification is also important during summer months. But, in the process, you can lose vital nutrients which need to be replaced. For example, the key mineral magnesium can be lost by sweating and during exercise. This may not seem all that important until you realize that magnesium is required to monitor heart rate, blood pressure, blood vessel constriction, muscular contraction and is a component of over 300 chemical processes in the body. It's also critical that calcium is balanced with magnesium. A lack of nutritional magnesium (which is required daily) and an excess of calcium can lead to a host of symptoms ranging from low energy and fatigue, to constipation, muscle cramps, spasms or tics, rapid heart rate, PMS, shortness of breath and a number of more serious conditions.

Good health starts at the cellular level. Cells (an estimated ten trillion in a human body) are the building blocks of life. In order for your body to be in top shape, all the cells that compose your body have to be healthy.

ELECTROLYTES (MINERALS)

I've been taking saunas for many years for maintenance detoxification and to keep my skin looking young. While in the sauna I take electrolytes as they get sweated out. The electrolytes are magnesium, potassium, sodium and calcium. If those electrolytes are not replaced, deficiencies of them will cause all sorts of mild to severe heat-exhaustion symptoms. It's the same if you live in a hot, humid area of the country, if you do physical labor outside or even while spending time in the garden during a warm or hot afternoon. The body *must* have electrolytes to survive hot climates.

Remember, sweating is the body's natural method of cooling off. If you're not drinking enough water, you won't sweat. So if you find yourself hot or not sweating while in the sauna or out in hot weather, go somewhere to cool off, drink enough water and take enough minerals until you feel re-energized. It's just *amazing* how many people are mineral-deficient and dehydrated. Those two factors alone can account for the majority of health problems.

Here's a very useful tip: A friend of mine who was raised in South Africa told me about something she does for fatigue due to hot weather. Lemons contain most, if not all, the minerals a body needs. Cut a lemon (organic if possible) into quarters, take one or more of the quarters, sprinkle it with iodized sea salt (available at your health food store) and suck the juice out of it. You'll feel better right away if you're over-heated. Water with a small amount of lemon juice is also an excellent way to get minerals.

TRACE MINERALS

Trace minerals, also known as trace elements, are required daily in very small amounts for good health and beautiful hair. These include minerals like: boron, chromium, copper, manganese, molybdenum, selenium, silicon, sulphur, iron, cobalt, iodine and zinc. There are too many of them to list here but know that a complete liquid ionic trace mineral supplement is essential. You can also find trace minerals in tablets that break down easily.

There are minerals and there are trace minerals. The essential minerals the body needs are calcium, sodium, magnesium and potassium. Trace minerals are those minerals required by the body in trace (very small) amounts. Without all of these minerals, nothing in the body works correctly. Chapters could be written on their value. A trace mineral supplement whether by pill or liquid, generally contains all the trace minerals.

To be certain you're taking the correct balance of vitamins, minerals and trace minerals your body needs, it's very smart to see a competent nutritionist.

To recap:

a. Take the basic live vitamins: A, B, C, D, and E

b. Ensure you get the required daily amount of calcium, magnesium, potassium and sodium

c. Take your liquid ionic trace minerals

...all in the proper balance.

Excellent nutrition is the foundation for beautiful hair. Vitamins, minerals and trace minerals give the hair follicles what they need to help grow beautiful hair. This is basic and essential.

See the "Products" section at www.themodernrapunzel.com for live vitamins and minerals.

Remember anytime you're considering supplementation, be sure to maintain as healthy a lifestyle as possible and follow the directions of the manufacturer or your natural-health practitioner carefully. This will ensure you give yourself the greatest probability of success in your supplement program. Remember, supplements are not enough on their own. One has to eat a healthy diet.

It's always the simple basics that work.

I hope this information has helped make the subject of vitamins and minerals clearer and has given you the direction to take to ensure your body is getting the supplementation it needs.

If you choose to grow a garden of your own, which is a very smart thing to do, you can read about a CD from a renowned expert on organic gardening made easy in the "Products" section on my website, www.themodernrapunzel.com.

Now I want to give you some real life examples of women who had hair loss and what they did to resolve it:

MINERALS

A woman was losing hair when she moved from Europe to the United States. The original Himalayan Crystal salt, full of minerals, stopped her hair loss. (Minerals from salt may be good for some and not for others. The point is to get an excellent source of minerals in your daily diet.)

PROTEIN

One woman was on a diet to handle another situation than hair loss and found she was grossly insufficient in protein. She began eating 60 grams of protein per day for her weight based on her doctor's recommendation. She started to see results in her hair growth within the first three weeks.

THYROID

A woman having trouble with her hair went to a nutritionist and found she was sensitive to wheat and gluten which had damaged her stomach lining. Those allergens caused her to not assimilate vitamins and minerals and interfered with her thyroid. She stopped eating anything with gluten in it, went on a nutritional program and her hair is great now.

VITAMINS

Another woman who had very thin hair did a custom vitamin program and now her hair is very thick.

JUICING

A woman told me she had been drinking sixteen ounces of a variety of vegetable juices daily for several months. As a result, her hair became even thicker than it was as a child.

LOW FAT DIET

A woman was on a very low-fat diet for two months and started losing hair. When she put the Omega 3, 6 & 9 oils back into her diet, she stopped losing her hair.

NUTRITION

A 54 year-old woman was losing her hair for no apparent reason. As a result of the correct nutritional program she not only grew back the hair she lost but it became thicker than before.

CANDIDA AND PARASITES

Another woman's hair was falling out by the handfuls due to a problem with candida and parasites. With a nutritionist's help her candida is gone, she regained her health and her hair became thicker than before.

NUTRA-SWEET

One woman was losing hair because of the Nutra-sweet in diet drinks.

For those of you whose hair is falling out, do not be overwhelmed by trying to figure out why it's happening. My intention is to give you the broad picture of health and nutrition, what can affect hair-growth and the vital role diet and correct supplementation plays in hair-loss.

By incorporating a healthy lifestyle and implementing the basics, health and hair-loss can turn around. An excellent nutritionist or natural health-care practitioner is worth his or her weight in gold.

Chiropractic

What does chiropractic have to do with a full and healthy head of hair? Everything! If the bones in the neck are out of alignment, the flow of blood and nourishment to the brain and scalp are inhibited.

What does chiropractic have to do with anti-aging? Everything! If the bones anywhere in the spine are out of alignment, the affected corresponding muscles, nerves and organs will do what's called atrophy (decrease in strength and size). Aches, pains and weakness in any part of the body make a person feel old. The easiest way to get immediate relief is to see a competent chiropractor.

An enormous beacon of light needs to be shone on the subject of chiropractic, spot-lighting it in its proper place in our world. But first, here's a little of my own background in relation to it so you understand why I'm so passionate about it:

I was a bit of a wild child in my younger years and managed to get myself thrown off horses once in awhile. I did silly things like jumping on a horse in a field without a saddle or bridle because my brother dared me to. The horse played his side of the game also, and promptly bucked me off. There were a few of those incidents until I learned to show the horse who's boss *with* a bridle! But it was all worth it.

Since when can we tell a child *and* an adult not to play, to live, to experience? Thank goodness there's a way to fix it! It's Chiropractic.

My own personal experience with chiropractors has shown me that *all* effective solutions are simple, basic and powerful. Without chiropractic, I would not have been able to accomplish what I have. Chiropractors are my heroes. They have helped me make my dreams come true.

As a result of the life-changing results I have received from these special, wonderful and expert beings, I decided to help them personally and professionally. I have worked with over 500 chiropractors one-on-one and in workshops for over fifteen years. I have learned so much about the profession, the quality of these beings who have made helping others their life's mission and the consistent miracles they perform on thousands of people on a daily basis.

Exercise

Oxygen is utilized in almost every function of the body. Exercise and breathing in oxygen revitalizes the whole body and carries the required nourishment to the cells of the scalp and face. A decrease in oxygen can cause anything from hair loss to unhealthy skin to fatigue to aging.

There is another vital reason to exercise. The breasts, especially towards the armpits, contain a large quantity of lymph glands which the body uses as a garbage-disposal unit to get rid of wastes and toxins within the body. The only way the lymph system can detoxify is through exercise, drinking water and massage.

The health benefits of daily exercise cannot be stressed enough. It promotes well-being, strengthens the immune system, maintains joint

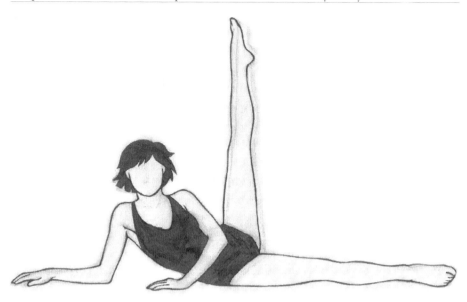

mobility, increases energy and the resultant increased blood circulation provides the scalp with nutrients and oxygen.

Look for opportunities all throughout your day to engage in physical activity.

WHAT SPECIFIC KIND OF EXERCISE SHOULD I DO?

Everyone does well with the kind of exercise they enjoy. Some like to lift weights, some like running, some like swimming, jumping on a mini-trampoline, dancing, walking, etc.

Rebounding on a mini-trampoline is one of the best exercises one can do with the least amount of effort. It helps every function in the body, naturally detoxifies and is great because, like the slant board, reverses the daily pull of gravity. As far as I'm concerned, it's the most health-giving of all the exercises. But then, it's my preference. Using a rebounder (mini-trampoline) for five minutes is equal to running a mile and helps build bone mass.

TAKING A WALK

A half-hour walk in the sunshine does two things:
1. The body absorbs vital vitamin D. Vitamin D helps with the process of calcium absorption.

2. Walking is the best exercise a person can do with the least stress on the body.

Cover your head with a hat or put a natural product on your hair that coats and protects it from the sun's heat. The sun's rays can be very damaging to hair.

BEST TECHNIQUE OF EXERCISING

My chiropractor told me the best technique of doing any kind of exercise.

Let's use the example of walking. He said: *"Walk at a brisk pace until you feel yourself getting a little tired, then continue walking but slow down for that same length of time. In other words, if you start to get a little tired in three minutes, slow down for three minutes until you have caught your breath and don't feel tired. Continue with that cycle as many times as you wish but remember, to get strong, one has to build up to it. If you feel you can only do one set of three minutes in a day, then that's all you should do. The next day try to do two sets of three minutes each. Gradually build up more and more of the three-minute sets until you know you're okay with increasing the time of each set."*

The kind of exercise best for you is the exercise you'll do because you enjoy it. It shouldn't be an ordeal. It should be a joy. Build up to a half an hour or hour every day. You're not only keeping the body functioning well, you're showing the body who's boss. It's always therapeutic to tell the body what to do.

Chapter Twelve

Toxic Load and Detoxification

Are you sick of hearing about toxins? I am. I'm sure for those of you who are health-oriented, you've read and heard about toxins a great deal.

It's important to understand how toxins affect the way we look and feel. For example, when the kidneys or liver are overloaded with toxins, one can get dark circles under the eyes. When one eats processed food, one's body becomes overweight, the hair loses its vitality, the eyes lose their gleam and the skin loses its natural healthy glow. When the intestines are overloaded, nutrients aren't absorbed, which means the cells aren't getting what they need. All of that leads to aging of the skin, hair and body. The list of observable and felt negative effects due to toxins goes on and on.

I've thought to myself: "Why can't the body just eliminate the toxins on an on-going basis instead of having to go through the agony of detoxification?"

Well, you can get the body to that point but it takes work. It's unfortunate we have detoxify at all, but the rewards are *well* worth the effort, even though it doesn't feel that way while going through it.

You're reading a book from a woman who, many years ago, was extreme with fasting. The pendulum couldn't have swung any further than what I put myself through. Now I know it was silly and unnecessary. If I added up all the weeks and months I fasted, it would amount to at least a year. Yes, I fasted on water, orange juice, grapes–the whole shebang.

At the time I thought that was the way to get healthy. I didn't know I was robbing my body of essential nutrients by long-term fasting. Now, I've come back to simple cleansing programs. The ideal cleansing program gives the body what it needs rather than one or two food items. Later on in this chapter are several painless and effective ways to cleanse the body of toxins.

Until our manufacturers take responsibility for synthetic body-care products, toxic household-cleaning products and all the rest of the poisonous substances put in and on our bodies, we will have to continue to cope with this injustice.

When we start demanding of our growers that they use only rich soil, rotate the crops and not use toxic pesticides and insecticides, we will then start to see a broad and dramatic change in health. In the meantime we have to deal with detoxification. I know it's not fair.

We *can* wake up the manufacturers and growers through an uncompromising insistence of our inherent rights. We can start by purchasing natural and organic products only.

> *"As caretakers of life we affect the balance of nature to such a degree that our own actions determine whether the great cycles of nature bring prosperity or disaster. Our present world is the unfoldment of a pattern we set in motion."*
> **The Balance of Life – Hopi Prophecy**

I DON'T RECALL GIVING ANYONE THE TITLE TO MY BODY

Have you watched the TV ads advertising the latest pharmaceutical (drug or medicine)? Such and such relieves heartburn. But, in a very subdued voice, while at the same time watching the "happy" woman with no heartburn, comes the truth–the side effects!

Don't most of the side effects sound a heck of a lot worse than the original problem the person had? How many people do you know would prefer to substitute heartburn with diarrhea, vomiting, headaches and nausea?

The ad *should* say "Pick your symptoms! Choose from heartburn or diarrhea, vomiting, headaches, nausea!" Please excuse me for getting sarcastic. It's appalling.

Have you seen the physician's manuals on pharmaceuticals and their side effects? First, there's the name. And then for anywhere from half a column to sometimes several columns or pages long are listed the side effects.

Of course not everyone will experience side effects. But do you think it's possible side effects are a sign there might be something inherently wrong with the "solution"? We can blindly accept those solutions without inspection and accept the side effects as "normal." They're not.

Some of the psychotropic drug (affecting the mind or mood) side-effects include suicide. It doesn't make for fun reading.

Any symptom one is trying to eliminate with a pharmaceutical solution may cause more problems than they solve as witnessed by the extensive list of side effects. As you've seen in the TV ads, the "solution" can show up later in other symptoms caused by the drug. Who knows how many drugs and their side effects can cause major problems with hair and skin?

Many physical problems are often the early warning signs of nutrition-related disorders. Handling physical symptoms with temporary "band-aids" (as in pain medication) may prolong the healing process by not getting to the real cause.

Please understand that I am *not* telling you to go off your medications or drugs. That is between you and your doctor. Talk to him or her. Get more information; the information you need to make the right decision. Some medications are essential for life. I want to be very clear about that. But to indiscriminately depend on them as the solution to all ills invalidates the innate healing abilities of Mother Nature.

There are natural alternatives for every condition, ones that won't cause side effects, from natural sleep aids to remedies for indigestion to herbs for depression, etc., etc. Mother Nature has provided us with hundreds of powerful healing herbs and natural remedies. They may not solve every single problem but it's worth giving them a try first. Another benefit is that in many cases, if not most cases, the natural remedies are *much* less expensive.

When I was nineteen, the year of my Wake-Up Call, I ran a medical doctor's office. I knew nothing about health.

One day a representative from a pharmaceutical company came to visit the doctor I was working for. (I will call the doctor "Dr. J.") Unbeknownst to the representative and Dr. J, I overheard a conversation they were having behind "closed doors," except the door was still open a crack. I listened. The representative told Dr. J about a particular medication that hadn't been thoroughly tested out yet and would like Dr. J to test it on his patients and report back to him. Something smelled unethical to me. But what did I know?

Dr. J started prescribing the untested medication to many patients. I didn't know what ailment it was intended to handle but I do know that all of a sudden patients were coming in sicker from the drug than they were from whatever ailment they had. It was appalling to watch.

By then I was starting to get a real, honest-to-goodness clue that something was amiss in Doctor-J-land.

I am not indicating that most, or any medical doctors in this day and age are unethical. But that experience planted the seeds of my "Wake-Up Call." I quit and never looked back.

The natural health industry is booming.

That's a very good thing.

Protect your health and well-being by becoming fully informed and educated on what you put into your body.

The Effects of Toxins in the Body

The following is vital information about the body obtained from Dr. Ian Shillington, a noted Naturopath.

THE BRAIN

The most important organ in the entire body is the pituitary gland located in the back central part of the brain. This organ is responsible for keeping us fit and young, and is also the communication center that gives orders to all the other glands and pushes them to do their jobs. It is the "Command Center" for the entire human body.

If you know of someone suffering from Alzheimer's or Parkinson's Disease, it's because of difficulties in the brain. Most people are not aware that overweight issues also have a direct correlation to the pituitary gland. There are herbs that feed the cell structures of the brain, increase circulation to the whole area and cleanse the brain cells by unclogging blood vessels within. These herbs are gingko biloba, gota kola, kola nut, calumus and rosemary which can kick-start an almost non-functional pituitary gland.

THE LIVER

The next most important organ in the body is the liver. This is the organ that corrects and detoxifies all of the organs and glands in the body. It is the only organ that contributes to keeping the pituitary in good shape. When the body has to deal with toxic-laden foods day after day, the liver gets to a point where it is just too busy trying to survive on its own and no longer has the ability to correct all the other organs and glands in the body which is supposed to be its main job. The next thing you know you're sick with one or more of a thousand diseases.

THE KIDNEYS

Dr. Shillington states the importance of keeping the kidneys clean of waste. The kidneys have several functions, the most important being the removal of wastes and toxic substances from the body.

He says that by continuing to eat commercial foods day after day, foods that contain pesticides and other toxins, brings the kidneys to a point where they no longer have the ability to do their job; the job of filtering toxic substances out of the body. The next thing that happens is the body becomes sluggish and one's energy level goes down. Kidney stones may develop or some other kidney problem shows up, manifested as one or more of a hundred different disease symptoms in the body.

It is essential to do intestinal, liver and kidney cleanses. If you don't change the oil filter in your car once in awhile, it gets sluggish and eventually will quit. It's the same with the eliminative organs. If any of these organs are blocked, the body cannot perform its normal functions. Disease and aging result.

See the "Products" section at www.themodernrapunzel.com for intestinal, liver and kidney cleanses.

MEDICINES AND DRUGS

Drugs are a temporary solution with resultant long-term problems. The natural method provides a predictable and stable means of restoring health fully. Work with your doctor to be able to wean off any unnecessary medications or drugs. Some are required to sustain life, but many are not. Some are life-saving on a short-term basis. One has to have and use judgment. Ask questions. Get reliable information and act accordingly.

INDOOR AIR POLLUTION

Neither state nor federal governments regulate indoor air pollution and how toxic household products might affect the air inside our homes. Chemical products are used in most households on a daily basis; everything from general cleaners for surfaces and windows, bleach, laundry detergent with fragrance, fabric softeners, etc.

Many of the symptoms of depression and hyper-activity come from allergic reactions to these common products. Even when the containers are closed, they can have a tendency to "out-gas," meaning the fumes from the products permeate the air. Then you and your loved ones breathe them.

Dump those household toxic chemical cleaners and products. All of them! And not down the drain as it will further pollute the water system.

USE SAFE PRODUCTS

In today's world, the incidence of exposure to unnecessary toxic substances is substantial: air and water pollution; pervasive chemical use (the average household contains 63 different dangerous chemicals for a total of approximately 10 gallons of hazardous chemicals); insecticides; pesticides; excessive use of sugar; processed foods; drugs and medicines.

Poisons weigh down on the body and affect us spiritually, being connected with bodies that we are.

There are many excellent non-toxic products available to clean with. For example, one of the best ways to cut grease on surfaces and clean glass is diluted white vinegar in a spray bottle. It's as good if not better than popular window-cleaning products, which are horrendously toxic.

Peroxide is amazing for disinfecting. Just make sure it's used only on surfaces (like sinks) that won't be affected by its bleaching action. I put my toothbrush in the peroxide bottle to disinfect it. Then, without rinsing the peroxide off the toothbrush, brush my teeth.

Never use chlorine bleach for anything as the chlorine vapor can damage the lungs.

Check the labels. Choose fragrance-free items. Don't pick chemical anti-bacterial soaps. Pick laundry detergent based on natural disinfectants such as eucalyptus, tea tree oil, rosemary or sage plant rather than petroleum.

I could tell you many stories about the harmful effects of popular laundry detergents and fabric softeners. But I'll tell you one. A family member of mine was having headaches for years. He tried every remedy he could think of and nothing helped. And then I mentioned to him to try changing his laundry detergent and fabric softener to a natural one to see what happened. Voilà! *No more headaches!* And I could finally breathe around him.

Never use synthetic perfumes or cologne. They are more damaging than you can possibly imagine, and they affect those in the surrounding environment who are allergic to them. Severe chemical sensitivities to artificial fragrances are becoming more and more widespread.

There are harmless, natural products for *every use* and wonderful plant-based perfumes to be found at your health-food store.

Please save yourself and those you love from environmental toxins.

See the "Products" section at www.themodernrapunzel.com for safe and effective cleaning products.

SHALL WE CREATE A SAFE ENVIRONMENT, INSIDE AND OUT?

If we do anything Mother Nature doesn't do, there's trouble. Would Mother Nature put toxins in her soil, in her air, in our bodies? No. Toxins defeat nature's ability to heal and beautify naturally.

The body defends itself by storing toxins as best it can. At the point it can no longer store them it will start dumping those toxins into the system. And then we don't feel so good, to put it mildly.

Our awareness has gradually moved away from the basic, workable ways of taking care of ourselves to that of a chemical world. Our natural defense systems have become over-loaded and put strain on even Mother

Nature's ability to deal with the onslaught of poisons. What is a poison? It's anything Mother Nature didn't create in its pure state.

Premature aging of the body is just cumulative toxins, lack of proper nutrition and stress. Isn't that interesting? That's it, the *only* reasons!

Detoxification is a vital process that many people don't really understand. It's the process of cleaning out of the body any substances that shouldn't be there or aren't needed. When unnecessary substances invade the body, they must be collected and removed. Otherwise they will be stored, which opens the door to illness and degenerative diseases.

It's important to understand that the physical, mental and spiritual all work together. Each one enhances or detracts from the other according to the condition of the other two. Being connected to a body with poisons inhibits one's mental and spiritual expression.

Continued headaches, constipation, brain fog, fatigue, irritability, aches, pains, unhealthy skin and hair, to name *just a few* of the signs of toxicity, can be very discouraging. These symptoms oftentimes change our whole attitude towards life and may leave us desperately seeking solutions without relief. Resorting to pain killers and unnecessary drugs only compounds the problem because one's overall health continues to take a dive. In some cases that downward spiral can make us want to give up which is not okay and not necessary.

Let's put a halt to that dwindling spiral, or at least slow it down enough for the time being to gain some real hope and experience positive change. Then you'll have enough certainty to take the healing process all the way home.

How Does One Painlessly Detoxify?

ENEMAS

Ew! How disgusting! The "E" word may be as unpleasant to you as a four-letter word. You might be asking yourself, "Do I even want to read about this?"

Let me see if I can talk you into it.

Enemas not only give great overall relief but help one look and feel much younger. The skin clears up and takes on a nice, healthy glow, the eyes start to sparkle again, the face has fewer wrinkles, hair growth is assisted considerably and you and your body have more energy! What's that worth?

We don't need to go over the percentage of people, especially in this country who are sick. There's no point in elaborating on it. If you're reading this book, I'm sure you already know or have heard. Well, how are we going to make up the damage and achieve vibrant health? You gotta clean house first, so you can re-decorate.

May I be candid? Is there any other way?

I don't even know where to begin on the positive changes that result when old, decaying, putrefying poop has been removed from one's intestines.

The cells in your body receive nutrition from the food you eat. That food has to pass through the intestines. If the intestines are clogged, your body will absorb less nutrition. And guess what? You're hungry! The body wants nutrition. And so does your scalp and hair.

Hunger is the body's mechanism telling you it needs nutrition. You eat more to satisfy the hunger but the nutrition can't get to the cells. Weight continues to accumulate with no real relief in hunger. It's a vicious cycle.

Let me start first by saying that if you want to look and feel a whole heck of a lot younger and lose weight, I mean *a whole heck of a lot younger and lose weight*, then you'll consider taking the plunge (pun intended).

Silent-film star Mae West's secret to beauty was colonics. (Those are enemas administered by a trained practitioner.)

Here is my personal story.

Many years ago, I was pushing my body way beyond what it could cope with and I wasn't taking the usual good care of myself. I was starting to look my age. Vain as I was (and still am, and proud of it), I had to do something fast. I found a knowledgeable nutritionist who told me to take daily enemas until the stress on the body was relieved. Being in the kind of position I was in, I was willing to do whatever it took. I did the enemas, got on the right diet and took the right supplements, all at the same time.

During this undignified process of daily enemas, I noticed something truly amazing. After not looking in the mirror for a few days, I then got my courage up and gave my face a glance. I stopped in my tracks and slid back to the mirror. My face was starting to markedly de-age! Wrinkles were disappearing, my eyes were getting back their sparkle, the puffiness under my eyes was disappearing, my skin color had a nice natural glow and my hair was starting to have a healthy shine again. Whoa! The sacrifice of my dignity was paying off!

What a woman will do to look her best!

I would never have known what this process of enemas could do until I went through it myself. It didn't take long and I knew when I was done with the process. My body felt light as a feather and I knew the nutritious foods and supplements I was taking were being fully assimilated.

Here's another short story to illustrate just how bad it can get.

Believe it or not there was a woman who had barely gone to the bathroom for a year. She finally went on intestinal cleansing tablets for a month. And still nothing. Five weeks into it, she started to poop and pooped for three days straight. She lost some huge amount of weight in those three days.

It's pretty scary to know that a majority of the unnecessary weight that bodies carry around is poop. Look at anyone with a paunch and know that it's mostly that "stuff."

Do you want to lose weight, detoxify your body and feel and look a whole lot better? Do enemas and colon cleanses. But do them correctly and safely.

If you're stand-offish about doing it yourself, there are colon therapists you can go to. Let them do the dirty work. They're used to it. I've used them. And it's fun to laugh with them about the whole thing.

Remember to replace the good bacteria in the intestines with acidophilus. There are many good brands in your local health-food store.

Do you still love me?

Well, let me make it up to you. Here's what you can do in addition to taking enemas or if you just can't face doing enemas at all:

1. Take an intestinal cleansing product.

See the Products section at www.themodernrapunzel.com for a gentle and effective intestinal cleansing product.

2. Gradually switch from processed foods to nothing but whole organic foods.

3. The lymphatic system is the drainage system of the body. It does not operate on its own. There are only three ways it will function: exercise, water and massage. Find the kind of exercise you like. Indulge yourself in massage when you can. Both massage and exercise get the circulation going to help the cells release toxins. Be sure to drink plenty of water after both. As a side note: Bob Hope's secret to long life was a daily massage. He lived to be a hundred years old.

4. Make your home environmentally safe. Get rid of all the chemicals in the house and replace them with all-natural cleaners.

5. Water. Drink your quota.

6. Vegetable juice! It's vital to give the body the nutrients it needs while undergoing a cleansing program and in general. There's no better source of nutrients than fresh, organic vegetable juices. They also assist in the detoxification process.

7. Saunas. As mentioned earlier, the skin is the largest eliminative organ there is. Toxins pour out of the skin while sweating in a sauna. The toxic load taken off the body from doing saunas is just incredible. Plus it makes your face look years younger.

I may sound like a broken record, but again remember to consume *plenty* of water and minerals while sweating. Salt, potassium and magnesium are sweated out during a sauna or exercise and it is *vital* they be replaced. By taking these extra minerals while in the sauna and *whenever* your body is sweating, you're preventing heat exhaustion symptoms and protecting your cells.

There are some wonderful powdered electrolytes to put in water to drink while in the sauna. One is "Emergen-C" available in packets from the health food store. Another great way to get minerals is homeopathic cell salts and salt and potassium tablets generally in the ratio of one salt to two potassium. (If you have high blood pressure, check with your doctor first to determine whether it's safe for you to take saunas, salt and potassium.) Take as many doses as needed depending on how long you're sweating. If you don't take in enough minerals and water, you will be exhausted. You should feel relaxed and rejuvenated after a sauna, definitely not depleted.

8. Foot Bath. It's one of the easiest ways to rid the body of accumulated toxins quickly. Believe it or not, it's a special machine that pulls and eliminates toxins from every organ in the body and the lymph, through the feet. It's completely safe if you follow instructions. It can also help rid the body of toxic metals which are responsible for many major health problems. You actually see the toxins come out in the water as you're taking a foot bath. It's remarkable. Some chiropractors have them in their offices.

See the "Products" section at www.themodernrapunzel.com for a foot bath.

9. Liquid Zeolite. This is a product taken orally in water that captures toxins and eliminates them through the elimination system. More and more people are experiencing enormous relief and benefit from taking this product.

See the "Products" section at www.themodernrapunzel.com for liquid zeolite.

10. Foot pads. These are pads you put on your feet right before bed and sleep with them all night. The ingredients in them pull toxins out of the body through the feet. They work great.

See the "Products" section at www.themodernrapunzel.com for foot pads.

11. Once you're up to it, clean the bowel, liver and kidneys through a specific detoxification program.

It's more than likely you'll have some accompanying symptoms during this process. How you feel and look may get worse before it gets better, but you're definitely getting better as long as you continue. Slow down the process if it's too difficult. Proceed gently so the body has a chance to get used to it. Ensure you work closely with a health practitioner.

And last, here is a simple action that makes the process of detoxification much easier:

12. Activated charcoal capsules and barley tablets or powder obtained from your health-food store. These tablets absorb toxins before they can enter your bloodstream. Take five to fifteen tablets of each, together with eight ounces of water as many times a day as needed. I take them for a quick detox whenever I need to; when I've been exposed to toxins in the environment or if I'm feeling a little "out of it." They also assist in the healing process during a cold, flu or any illness. You can also take them after a sauna to absorb the toxins. Don't be surprised when discovering your stool is black. It's the charcoal.

Toxins are acidic and as mentioned before an acid system is a key contributor to hair-loss. An acidic condition also makes a person grouchy. One or more of these procedures will help alleviate the acidic condition, calm the body and make life much, much easier on you and those you love. The only way you'll know the difference is in recognizing how you felt before as compared to after. If this sounds like a lot, it could be harder.

These are methods that substantially shorten the detoxification and healing process, especially enemas, saunas, liquid zeolite and foot baths.

As you start implementing one or more of these procedures, you'll notice your hair will start to regain its natural beauty, your energy will start returning, your eyes will be brighter and clearer, you'll have a bounce in your step and a new outlook on life, for real.

Again, I recommend being under a natural doctor's care while undergoing any detoxification program.

To recap:

1. Enemas.
2. Take an intestinal cleansing product.
3. Gradually switch from processed foods to nothing but whole organic foods.
4. Water, exercise and massage.
5. Make your environment environmentally safe. Get rid of all the chemicals in your house and replace them with all-natural products.
6. Water. Drink your quota.

7. Vegetable juice.

8. Saunas.

9. Liquid zeolite.

10. Foot Bath.

11. Foot pads.

12. Clean the bowel, liver and kidneys, in that order, through a specific detoxification program. Ensure you work closely with a health practitioner.

13. Activated charcoal and barley tablets.

I wish you the *very best of luck* with whichever detoxification program you and your natural health-care practitioner decide on. Any and all of these procedures noticeably facilitate the detoxification process.

And now, here is the chapter devoted to helping you lighten the load of daily living: The Factors of Stress and Hair Loss.

Chapter Thirteen

The Factors of Stress and Hair Loss

Stress in any form leads to depletion of body and soul. Stress is more a factor in hair loss than most people realize, which is why I have included so much on the subject of stress in this book. When a person's stress level diminishes, nutrition starts to take hold. Real healing and positive change can then occur. The happier one is, the more one's body cooperates.

What impact does stress have on our health and our hair? Huge. Hair loss is epidemic; not just for men but women also. Hair loss in women is not known of widely, as it's not openly talked about. But when we look at the day-to-day demands put on women in this day and age, it makes sense.

When I was growing up, most women were full-time mothers. Now, most women, in addition to being mothers, work full-time jobs. A lot of women are single moms. They're exhausted. And then there's what's in the news, the ex-husband, being overweight, and, and, and... enough already!

We all know trying to survive in this high-paced world is a challenge. But "survival" is not good enough. How do we not only rise to the energy required by day-to-day activities, but other things that are important to us? The number one complaint in America is "I'm tired."

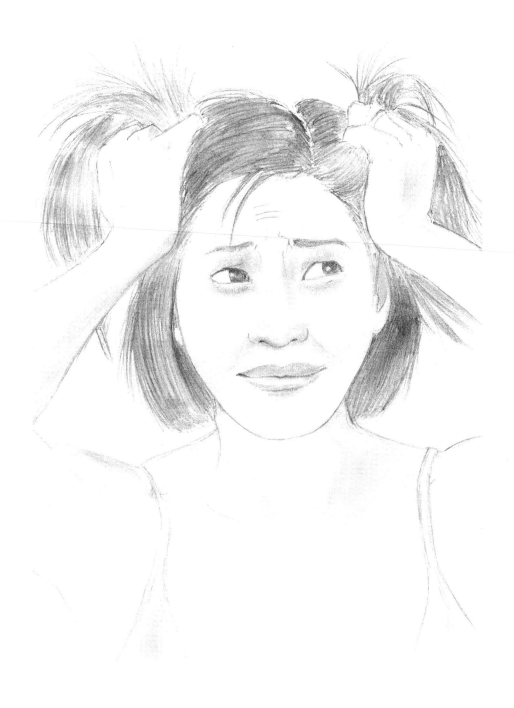

When we're stressed, the scalp gets tight making it difficult to grow new hair, the hair has a tendency to gray, look limp and lose its shine as stress is using up vital nutrients in the body. Hair can then fall out in small or large amounts, the face shows major signs of stress in the skin's overall color, texture and resiliency, not to mention wrinkles from scowling! Stress takes the #1 toll on the body, which of course dramatically affects how we look and feel.

Mental stress will rob the body of nutrients more than any other single factor there is. Second is chemical stress: toxins in our food and chemical body-care products, environmental pollutants, drugs and alcohol. Third is from physical pain and discomfort. Sometimes it gets very confusing to isolate which of these influence our ability to become truly strong and healthy.

Let's take up the body first.

PHYSICAL STRESS

So much of this book is what to do to: a) lighten the load of the adverse effects the body has upon you, b) help you achieve the goal of looking and feeling the way you want to and, c) provide you with answers that consult your common sense so you can do what is meaningful to you.

Simplicity and the basics are the whole emphasis and essence of this information. Let's move in the direction of "underwhelming" ourselves, instead of more overwhelm. I'm sure we can agree on that.

Okay. When *you* are under stress, the body can become the negative effect of that stress. It's safe to say that's the case with most, if not all people. The body will burn up nutrients in relation to one's activity level and how much negativity one is dealing with in life.

One of the unfortunate side effects of too much stress is hair loss and aging skin. The body just doesn't have enough energy to maintain hair growth and nourish the skin. It has more "important" (I'm sure those who are losing their hair will disagree) functions to perform, like keeping the heart beating and breathing.

As we've gone over in the section on diet and vitamins, there are basic needs of the body. Well, under stress or high activity, the body needs more, *a lot more,* of those fundamentals in relationship to what's happening.

The stress supplements are mostly the B vitamins. B vitamins are also known as the hair vitamins. Adding more B vitamins, natural not synthetic, to your supplement intake during demanding times will help you weather stress and will help prevent hair loss.

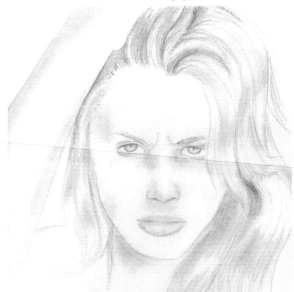

The other essential supplement to take during times of stress is *calcium*! There are seven kinds of calcium. Yes, seven! Calcium is *vital* for *all* functions of the body, especially the key organ, the liver, in handling stress. Vitamin D helps absorb calcium so remember this important vitamin too.

Talk to your nutritionist. Get the right balance of vitamins and minerals you need to go along with the increase.

It's essential to maintain an excellent diet while under any kind of stress. It's easy to hit the cookie jar or order pizza while under stress but do your best to stay away from nutrient-deficient foods, especially anything with sugar in it. Sugar makes it more difficult to weather tough times as it compounds the physical depletion one experiences during stressful times. Even though sugar is a great comfort food, you'll get through stressful times much easier and faster without it.

Very small amounts of high-quality protein a few times a day is especially essential. It gives the body strength to help weather the emotional and physical storms as protein doesn't burn up quickly.

RESERVES

Have you heard the term "reserve energy"? Hardly anyone has heard of it because they don't *have any*! That means "energy that's not already burned up." We need lots of reserve energy, not only to sustain day-to-day living but to have plenty for *fun*!

You may say, "Fun? What's that?"—My point exactly.

Negative emotion, which is the indicator of stress, takes its toll. The body inevitably becomes the recipient of that negative emotion which shows up in how we look and feel.

Chronic stress weakens the immune system and ages the body. When the body has to continually try to repair itself due to the on-going wear and tear of stress, it gets tired. As a result it isn't able to stabilize and replenish itself the way it normally can.

The body stores whatever resources it can during the good times for use during the stressful times. During times of increased stress, the body will draw upon whatever stored-up nutrients it has. If there aren't enough reserves to weather the difficult times, the body will start to degenerate as it has nothing to draw from. There's no reserve energy. Then one can become *very* tired and it will take time to recuperate. During those times, you may also notice an increase in hair loss.

Now is the time to make a decision, a decision in your own words, made to yourself. Your positive attitude about the healing process is your number one asset to utilize. I know this can be hard to do while under stress, but it's vital to have an up-beat attitude to facilitate healing. There are tools coming up to help you acquire and nurture that up-beat attitude, but your decision to succeed is where your healing begins.

So, if you would like to be able to deal with stress and have fun, no matter what is going on in life, *up the quality* (not quantity) of the nutrient-rich foods you're eating and *up the quantity* of supplements. You'll be able to deal with stress much more effectively.

MENTAL STRESS:

An article in the Vocational Educational Journal reported that 75-90 percent of the visits to doctors are stress-related. That's a huge percentage, wouldn't you say?

Like certain books and movies, stress has been at the top of the "best seller" list for a long time. Its effect on health and beauty is enormous.

There are those who make a living off others remaining stressed, the evening news broadcasters for one. I'll let you think of others.

I've tried to make you laugh during this book and not take things so seriously. But how easy is it to be light-hearted when we listen to the news every night? Make I make a suggestion? Throw rotten eggs at the screen or whatever. Just turn it off!

Which is better; to fall asleep with nothing on your mind or the latest horror-story you just heard on late-night news? So what, if you're not "in tune" with local and world events! What's more important: your sanity, or sounding smart at the office when everyone is giving their opinion on this or that crisis? I hope you answered, "My sanity."

One of my best friends gives me a synopsis about twice a month on what's going on so I don't sound like a complete idiot when someone brings up "something important." It's kind of useless though, because as soon as she tells me, it goes in one ear and out the other. So, big deal if I sound like an idiot when I say, "What terrorist"?

It's not that I don't care. It's just that I have more important things to do—like help people.

Anything you find draining, exhausting or upsetting, get it out of your life. And that doesn't mean your family or best friends. They're different.

We get what we put our attention on. And that's not just a handy little cliché. It's so true. It's not just *where* we put our attention, it's *what* we put our attention on. TV shoot-em-ups ain't it, late-night news ain't it, those disgusting terrorists ain't it. (See? I put your attention on the terrorists. Now you're thinking about them. See what I mean?)

We've all heard of "collective consciousness." If we all shifted our attention to what we *really* want, instead of the apparent ugliness in the world, we would see a *dramatic shift* in the well-being of this world we live in. *Please take this to heart.*

STRESS "HANDLINGS"

Seventeen million or more children and adults worldwide are on psychotropic drugs, ten million in the US alone!

Our parents weren't put on psychotropic drugs, nor were our grandparents. Why do you think that is? Could it be because of the overall quality of their diet and quantity of environmental pollution was entirely different then compared to now? Look at it. Doesn't it make sense? How could all these mental problems crop up, if they're not manufactured by these horrific causes?

In this complex world we tend to not even consider simple solutions. That's why things are complicated. We think in order for things to be the way we want, it requires a great deal of thought. All we have to do is look and see what has changed from the better to know what's happening. Let's go back to what's worked. The hardest and most complicated thing in life is getting others to see how simple things really are. All one has to do is look.

Our mental health depends on what we allow our attention to focus on. Some say it's much easier said than done to stay positive and enjoy life, but is there any other way you know of to bring about sanity and happiness for yourself and those you love?

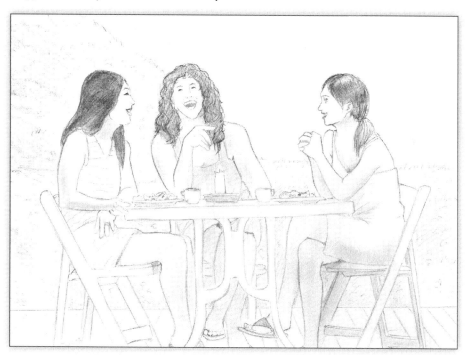

Let me share an excerpt from the article Survival Value by Elbert Hubbard, one of the greatest visionaries of all time, circa 1915. He gives us the core viewpoint on living a simple, fulfilling life.

Actions have survival value according to the degree of good that grows out of them...

All worthy deeds, all honest work, all sincere expressions of truth—whether by pen or by voice—have a survival value. Civilization is a great, moving mass of survival values, augmented, increased, bettered, refined, by every worthy life...

Hate, revenge, jealousy, doubt, negation, have no survival value.

Courtesy, kindness, good-will, right intent, all add up to the sum of human happiness. Not only do they benefit the individual who gives them out, but they survive in various forms and add to the well-being of the world.

All acts, whether work or play, should be judged with the idea of survival value in mind...

The reading of good books has a survival value. Games played in the open air have a survival value. Anything that gets you out in the sunshine, takes you across fields, out under the blue sky, has a survival value.

There is something about getting on good terms with the out-of-doors, with the soil, the trees, the plants, the birds, the flowers, that is great gain...

Anything that brings men together so they talk, read, think, laugh, play, makes them better men. These things stand for fellowship...

"Through language we touch finger-tips with the noble, the great, the good, the competent, living or dead, and thus are we made brothers to all those who make up the sum-total of civilization."

HOW DO WE MAKE OUR LIVES WHOLE?

Ultimately each and every source of stress we face in life challenges our body's ability to maintain its core strength: the strength needed to support and maintain basic functions, like hair growth. Because of this, it is vitally important to know how to manage stress in all areas of life.

We've covered how stress affects the health of your hair. Now there's the question of how to deal with stress; how you wish to change the way you look at things and restructure your life so you are empowered to apply the procedures.

The next section provides you, the whole woman, with enlightening solutions to the most common misconceptions, confusions and frustrations we face in life as women.

It is my genuine wish that the information and the inspirational quotes you are about to read will make a very noticeable difference in your life, your health and your happiness!

Part Two

You

The Whole Woman

Introduction

WHY IS IT THAT SO MANY WOMEN ARE LOSING THEIR HAIR?

And it's getting worse. I needed to reach deeper into the real causes beyond just the obvious ones.

I never thought I would write a book about hair loss. It took me years of personal trial and error to uncover the knowledge of what it takes to create a thick, gorgeous head of hair. As my hair grew thicker, longer and more beautiful, I changed. I changed because, all through my journey, I found basic truths about diet, about myself and my lifestyle. There were certain things I had to change to look the way I wanted and to become happy. I had many life-changing, personal realizations along the way.

Several years later I realized that thousands of women could physically, emotionally and spiritually benefit from what I have learned. Thus, this book was born.

Through embracing new and inspiring viewpoints that make complete sense to you, you will be empowered to follow your intuition by not compromising with your own truth.

Your overall well-being depends on it.

I quote best-selling author, Dr. Wayne Dyer, "*If you change the way you look at things, the things you look at change.*" Many small or large miracles can come out of changing your point of view.

My purpose in this section is threefold: 1) to present you with new viewpoints to consider, 2) to assist you with identifying some of the stress factors in your life and 3) to offer suggestions on what you can do to transform them into a win-win for you and everyone around you.

Some of the aspects of stress covered in this section may apply to you personally, some may not. Of those that do, the information and solutions given, when applied, will dramatically increase the effectiveness of the hair-growth procedures as laid out in this book. It's vital to bring relief from stress if we are to become healthy and happy.

It is my wish that you will have your own rewarding realizations while reading this section. The viewpoints and solutions revealed come from my own hard-won experience; what I have found to be true and what I have found that works. It there's anything that doesn't ring true to you, please reject it. What consults your understanding and your own reality is all that is important.

What's my passion? To do everything I can to help each woman gain certainty of her innate beauty and live her inner strength. Whatever I can do to assist her by facilitating her personal transformation from introversion to shining self-confidence, I will do. Period.

Let's throw caution to the wind and look at the last, but not least important part of our journey...

Chapter Fourteen

What is Beauty?

What has been considered beautiful down through the ages has changed. In different times and places an extra 50, 100, even 200 pounds was considered attractive.

Even in our own time the concept of beauty continually changes. Look at the phases of fashion and fads that vary from year to year that we women indulge in because it's fashionable–clothes, hair styles, makeup, etc, etc. This is not a bad thing. But who exactly are these trends set by? Do you know? I don't. It's a way of keeping markets changing in order to keep women buying. With that we're constantly trying to "fit in" and eventually, perhaps, but hopefully not, lose our own identity.

Let's get down to basics. Classic beauty withstands the test of time. It is a beauty that goes beyond fads. Beauty is being who you are—letting your own naturally-endowed physical and spiritual qualities (*and believe me, they're there!*) shine through without the blemish of anyone else's opinion of what is considered attractive or not.

The idea that only a few women are beautiful; that "only young women" or "actresses" or "those who have the right genes," etc., etc. are "endowed with this hard-to-capture quality" is false.

Every single woman is beautiful. Her innate beauty has always been there and always will be.

Beauty doesn't originate in a body. It originates in you; your decisions about it, letting it unfold and happen. I repeat – "because your innate beauty has always been there and always will be."

Beauty never goes away. It is nurtured to full expression.

I know a woman who didn't find her true beauty until 50 years old, the time of her life when she eliminated a major source of stress. She made a strong and courageous decision and as a result her natural beauty bloomed like the most exquisite flower you've ever seen. Her appearance before and after was dramatic. Before 50, she looked sad and haggard, her hair was drab and her skin was grey. After 50 her innate radiance began to shine through every pore of her body and her being. Her hair filled out dramatically and her skin took on a natural, radiant glow. She never went back on her decision and as a result her beauty continued to bloom.

It's truly amazing what stress will do to one's health and well-being and how much younger a person looks and feels after a source of stress is eliminated.

We all think stress is "normal." Well, it's not. It's common, not normal. Some think it's good to have stress in their lives as it keeps them motivated. Motivated to do what? I don't know, except perhaps motivated to avoid the source of the stress. Why can't we derive our motivation from our dreams and not from trying to avoid the pain? That's a good question to ask oneself when there's an internal debate going on.

Have you ever known a woman who made a big decision about her life: a change of career, a relationship, a move to somewhere else, changed her health habits, found her dream man, learned a new skill or followed her dreams, and then blossomed? Did you see her change from unhappy and "looking her age," to looking years younger? I've known women who have had that experience, including me.

The richness of a woman's physical and spiritual beauty comes to full expression through living by her true values without compromise. That's Ancient Beauty; everlasting.

Inner Beauty

You've heard a million times that inner beauty is real beauty. So the question is how to take that inner beauty and make it manifest? There's no trick, no mystery. It's simple. We're getting to that.

In some parts of the world women consider themselves beautiful no matter what. They have no burning need to show or prove anything.

In some countries, small breasts are considered sexy. There are hundreds of examples throughout the world of different ideas of what's considered beautiful and sexy. None of that matters.

You look beautiful because of your attitude. Your attitude about yourself is what defines who you are. What does that mean?

Let me give you some examples:

A person can emanate being "ugly" or being beautiful. A friend told me of a time when an overweight woman (by society's "standards") was standing behind him in a grocery store. When he turned to look at her, he flinched and thought to himself, "She's ugly!" Then he looked again. She was beautiful!

Because she was "overweight," she was putting out, like a flashing neon sign "I'm ugly!" She agreed to what this society considers ugly. It was a lie. Unfortunately the world will never see her as she really is because she agreed to that lie. My friend was smart enough to see through that.

Others will "get" how you perceive yourself. I have a male friend who was born with a cleft-palette. He was so self-conscious about it that his face would actually start to look deformed when he put his attention on it. He was causing it and of course my attention went to it. When his attention was not on it, he emanated self-confidence and his whole face changed.

He finally got the idea. I told him to put his attention on being his handsome self, instead of the cleft-palette. He hasn't talked about the cleft-palette in a long time. And boy is he handsome!

> *"Each person, each thing, has its special worth, which you must find and value. Cherish what is irreplaceable."*
> **From the book, "Ramses, The Son of Light"**
> **by Christian Jacq**

WHAT LIES BENEATH

I feel this story is deserving of its own special attention. It exemplifies the beauty of the human spirit.

One day, while living in San Francisco, I took the commuter train home known as "BART" (Bay Area Rapid Transit). The train was full of exhausted nine-to-five workers with glazed, passionless eyes. Most of them looked beaten by life, as in the line of the song "Old Man River"–"tired of living and feared of dying." I was getting ready to get on my inspirational soapbox when the train came to a stop, the doors opened and in popped a most amazing person!

Every person in the train was instantly stunned. His face looked like something out of a horror film; grotesque and almost unrecognizable as a human being.

Right away I recognized him as very special. Sensing that, he fell into the seat next to me with a beaming smile on his face. Every person in the train simultaneously and silently suppressed a huge gasp of horror and looked at me in panic, as if to say "What are you going to do?" I just sat there with a smile on my face, smug by not reacting. (My "inspirational talk" was now a silent one).

Thirty seconds later he reached his hand up to my head, ran it down my hair and said with genuine rapt admiration: "You have beautiful hair!" Another silent gasp of horror!

I turned and looked at *him*, not his face, and said straight to the being behind those eyes with recognition and appreciation from the bottom of my heart: "Thank you." At that moment I saw him move out to the size of the universe. He was an infinite, immortal being, not a body and he *knew it*! Someone had finally found, recognized and acknowledged him for the angel he was.

The train came to a stop. He jumped out of his seat, we looked at each other and smiled sweetly with our eyes. He bounded out the door.

I know he will never forget me as I will never forget him. In those two minutes between stops, we lived a lifetime. And the people in the train didn't know what happened; only that something did. I sat in my seat, not looking at anyone. I still felt every eye on me.

To this day, I hope the people in that train eventually "saw" what happened. If they did, they will never be just another face on a train, "tired of living and feared of dying." They will know to seek the magic in themselves and others, always.

> *"Beauty is not in the face; beauty is a light in the heart."*
> **Kahlil Gibran**

Chapter Fifteen

Your Individuality

Leaving Nothing for You

As women we naturally nurture others, but I have seen so many women fail to nurture themselves. Many women have told me of the stress in their lives due to primarily taking care of everyone else, leaving little to nothing for themselves.

How can a woman accomplish her dreams, be happy and have fun? How will she ever have enough energy to follow the procedures given in this book? She's being stretched too thin with too much to do! How can a woman continue to give and give without taking care of herself in the way she needs and wants to? She can't.

The saying "you have to love yourself" is so true. Through personal experience I've noticed that when I take care of myself first, I naturally help others also, as 1) I'm strong enough to do it and, 2) I'm helping from my own viewpoint, not from other "shoulds" imposed on me. This concept is one that may be met with disagreement, but if you want to look and feel great and be able to help others effectively, you'll consider yourself first.

A dear friend of mine told me recently, "The most important relationship I have is the relationship I have with myself." As a result it's easy to make the right decisions for all concerned. You first. Then you're strong enough for everyone else.

Another friend named Rivka has a very busy life. She has a husband who asks a lot of her, others who demand her time, has her own massage business, is a fundraiser for a major international project, is there to help her friends, create luscious meals and everything else attendant to life and living. But! She makes taking care of herself her first priority.

She never shows her face to the world until she's ready; until she's well-rested, feels and looks great. She doesn't do anything she doesn't want to do, including answering the phone. She elicits help from others to help her accomplish everything she wants in life. She's in control and it works. She leads an amazing, fulfilling life and so does everyone else around her. *Because of her, everyone wins.*

It took a long time for me to see that I have to take care of myself first. The concept challenged everything I've been taught. But I saw how Rivka's life works and I wanted that. So I made the decision and started taking control of what was important to me. As a result of that personal decision, I consistently implement what makes me look and feel great; the procedures and concepts in this book.

It's a juggle but eventually the rhythm starts happening and before you know it, you see genuine positive change in your life and those you love.

It's an exciting and challenging journey that will test your patience and persistence, but if you just keep taking care of yourself the way you want, before you know it everything lines up to you. That's a very, very worthwhile thing because a woman brings truth through living and expressing her innate integrity and wisdom.

Here's a man who is trying to tell us something vital:

> *"We're all here to help other people. That's the bottom line,*
> *but you have to help yourself first. Starting out in life, you're*
> *no good to anybody else unless you're good to yourself. If*
> *you're not healthy yourself you can't help anybody else."*
> **Bestselling author Matthew Lesko**

You're important. Treat yourself with unlimited respect and love. It's okay. Your well-being is as secure as you take care of yourself and have fun doing it. Being who you are and fulfilling your needs changes the world.

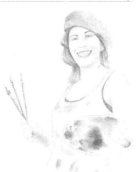

Please, my dear female friends, read this whole section on stress *at least twice*, first with the mind and second with the heart, until it's yours, until it makes complete sense to you, until you see for yourself what's worthwhile to you.

Anything that is truly important to you means you can do it no matter how "impossible" it may seem. The Soul of a Woman *requires* she let her true essence shine!

Brainwashing and Conditioning—All in One!

> *"Believe nothing, no matter where you read it or who has said it, not even if I have said it, unless it agrees with your own reason and your own common sense."*
>
> **Buddha**

Personal integrity is everything. What gets in the way of that?

The word "programming" also known as "brainwashing" and "conditioning" means the pressure of society of how we're supposed to look, how we're supposed to act, even how we're supposed to feel. We end up behaving in a certain way or thinking a certain way because it's "acceptable"?

There's nothing worse than not being able to be yourself.

Women are programmed to be sexy and look beautiful, otherwise "we're not accepted" or "desired by men." Spending your life trying to please others leaves nothing for you.

Create your own idea of how you'd like to look and feel. Otherwise it's like wearing 6-inch heels because your best friend wears them. Uncomfortable. Or maybe you'd like to wear 7-inch heels. It doesn't matter, as long as it's your choice.

Telling yourself "I'm beautiful" is not programming. Telling yourself you're beautiful is quite different than depending on what others say to determine how you feel about yourself.

Let me tell you a short story a male friend once told me. He met a woman who didn't fit the picture of what a beautiful woman "should" look like, but she always had an abundance of men competing for her attention. Why?

It's what she emanated. She saw herself, from her own viewpoint, as the most attractive woman in the world. And guess what? She was treated that way. She had no doubts about herself or her beauty.

Everyone is trying to figure out the magic formula, the magic pill, the magic! It's simple. Decide.

I can't tell you I don't wake up in the morning, look in the mirror and get upset or even a little depressed when I see aging signs. Instantly I change my attitude and decide "I'm beautiful," "I'm young." And then I forget about it and go about creating my life the way I want. As long as I'm doing that, I'm happy. And it shows.

You may be thinking, "Well, Miss Know-It-All—how can I be happy when I'm 25 (or more) pounds overweight?" I'm going to apologize even before I say this. What is so wrong about being 25 or more pounds overweight?

And now you're probably thinking, "What's *wrong* with her? Doesn't she *know*?" Yes, I do. That doesn't make you any less beautiful.

Have you ever noticed how hard it is to lose weight when you have to? When you're upset about it? Be kind to yourself. It will come off when you change your viewpoint. Much more on that coming up...

"Personality Types"

Please indulge me for a moment in my own hobby horse. "Personality Types" is a lie. *There is no such thing.* Every one of us is unique and cannot be put in a box to be compared or categorized with anyone else.

I know "Personality Types" is an attempt to explain human behavior. But the only way to explain human behavior is through the recognition that each and every person is very different and very special.

Now that we've established this, let's look at just *how special you really are*. Do you know you have unlimited power and ability? I would like to share a favorite quote of mine by Marianne Williamson. Here it is:

Our deepest fear is not that we are inadequate.
Our deepest fear is that we are powerful beyond measure.
It is our light, not our darkness

That most frightens us.
We ask ourselves,
Who am I to be brilliant, gorgeous, talented, fabulous?
Actually, who are you not to be?
You are a child of God.
Your playing small does not serve the world.
There is nothing enlightened about shrinking
So that other people won't feel insecure around you.
We are all meant to shine,
As children do.
We were born to make manifest
The glory of God that is within us.
It's not just in some of us, it's in everyone.
And as we let our own light shine,
We unconsciously give other people permission to do the same.
As we are liberated from our own fears,
Our presence automatically liberates others.

You'll never know how truly magnificent you are until you let your light shine. Who you really are is all your noteworthy qualities; unique to you, and only you.

The "Picture Theory"

One of my best friends, Marie, came up with this theory. I agree with it. See if you do.

We are continually bombarded with pictures of the "ideal" man or woman through movies, TV and magazines; the way they look, the way they act, who they are.

In relationships, one or both of the partners can be the unknowing victim of continuous comparison with those "ideals" by the other.

I give you this theory because a person can also do that to themselves; they impose on themselves their own "shoulds." They are comparing themselves against a picture of who they would like to be and what they would like to look like, whether that picture of their ideal comes from a movie, a magazine or a friend.

As a result, no matter how wonderful one is, one is never good enough because they "don't match up" to the picture created. Yes, created according to a model of some kind.

It's called the "Glamour Trap." If we're not aware of our agreement with it, we're consenting to the ultimate vicious trap. Yes, vicious is a strong word but appropriate. It's something we'll never be able to break unless it's looked at and evaluated according to the choices we make to create our own lives and happiness, from our own viewpoint.

Please my female friends, break the cycle of the "Glamour Trap."

The One and Only You

> *"I know what's it's like. I've seen it played out a zillion times. You're waiting for that magical day when someone makes the connection and recognizes who you really are. Maybe they'll first catch the sparkle in your eye. Or perhaps they'll marvel at your insights and the depth of your spirit. Someone who will help you connect the dots, believe in yourself, and make sense of it all. Someone who will understand you, approve of you, and unhesitatingly give you a leg up so that life can pluck your ready, ripened self from the branch of magnificence. Well. I'm here to tell you, your wait is over. That someone, is you."*

Mike Dooley, Author

Yes, you. Marvel in yourself.

Beauty is the expression of your natural qualities–your smile, your gestures, your flair, the way you carry yourself when you're self-confident and happy. It's your own style of clothes whether it's "in fashion" or not. It's because *you* love it! Twenty women can have twenty different ways of walking, talking and looking. They are all, every one of them, matchless.

Go with your own tastes. It's your individuality that speaks. Your likes and dislikes are your likes and dislikes. Why put yourself through doing something that isn't natural to you?

Not caring what others think of you, the way you act or the way you look, you'll be much happier, on your own path and have a great deal more self-confidence.

If wearing a purple scarf as a bracelet is how you want to express yourself, fantastic! It's an expression of you. You'll also be giving others permission to be themselves and license to express their own individuality.

Discover for yourself the effects you want to create upon the world. It is how you want to be seen and perceived while expressing your delicious self and living your dreams, as you.

How you project yourself is your calling card. It's how you're known.

Some days I feel like a cowgirl. That's how I dress on those days. Some days I feel like a princess. That's how I dress on those days. When I was working for a consulting company I broke the dress codes as much as I could get away with it. I always made sure I had my own individual flair no matter how I dressed.

Remember Rivka? She has all her clothes made just for her, even her shoes. Her clothes are made out of silk and velvet, tailor-made to her personality. She wears a different custom-made necklace every day. She wears flowers in her hair. Her "purse" is a small carrying basket. Her wallet is underneath fruit and flowers and she's always ready to give others one of her flowers or piece of fruit.

She may sound like a hippy. She's not. She never was. She is truly an individual. Everything about her is the manifestation of her own personality.

She is also the wisest woman I've ever known.

For years I laid on her massage table spilling my heart to her while her strong and gentle masseuse hands healed my body and her words soothed my soul. Her wisdom about women enlightened me, and her humor put my concerns in the proper perspective.

I, like many American women, had forgotten that I am a woman. But I *chose* to be a woman. I really *like* being a woman. But I thought I "should" be involved in the hustle-bustle of the business world, not above it.

It took years of Rivka's gentle coaxing that always, from the beginning, struck the bell of truth. But I wouldn't let the bell actually *ring* because of the pressures of the "shoulds." One day when she said firmly, "Jeanne! A woman's job is to bring beauty into the world!," the bell rang. At that moment I lost years off my face. I then began to be alert to and not agree with those ideas that weren't my own. I got off the treadmill long enough to look and listen to my own innate wisdom.

Without one's own personality being given full expression to, there's no sense of balance as individuals; we just have the material world. And that's not enough.

Beauty is sensual. It's essential. It's personal. It's spiritual. One of our roles is to endow life with inspiration, raising the human condition to the band of aesthetics.

When do you feel the best? Listening to your favorite music, looking at a beautiful sunset, doing all the things *you love* to bring out the essence of you

Whatever we can do as women to raise the environment to our highest of standards rather than let it dictate how we should feel and think, we will raise the whole sense of appreciation of life dramatically for ourselves and everyone we love. That's our job.

We are artists painting the palette of life. Be the real you. Not self-critical, but the one who doesn't care what anyone thinks, the one who is proud of herself for who she is. If you've lost that person, remember the last time you felt especially proud when you accomplished something you truly wanted to. That's you. Give it strength.

It's much more difficult to be "stressed out" when one has self-confidence.

Create the image in your mind that you're living the full expression of all your best qualities and abilities. Then bring it to life and delight in it! Being who you are and not following someone else's opinion of what you should be like, allows you to shine, really shine.

Your individuality is needed in this world. It's everything. Remember that always.

You *are* music. You *are* the sunset. *You are the beauty of mankind.*

> "*. . . . beauty is life when life unveils her holy face.*
> *But you are life and you are the veil.*
> *Beauty is eternity gazing at itself in a mirror.*
> *But you are eternity and you are the mirror.*"
> **Kahlil Gibran**

How Much Does the State of Mind Affect Appearance?

The answer is – dramatically! There's nothing more attractive than a man or a woman with self-confidence. One's posture, one's presence exudes a wavelength of beauty or ugliness or anything in-between. What you project gives other people the impression of who you are.

Have you ever heard the saying "Fake it until you make it"? What's wrong with standing up straight, (even if your body is overweight), walking proudly through a room and exuding a sense of self-confidence? Absolutely nothing. Keep doing it. Eventually you will truly feel it.

So now, how does one go about transforming a negative state of mind into a truly positive one so you don't have to continue to fake it? How do you discover your unique and wonderful qualities? How do you love yourself?

It's so easy to focus on physical qualities "considered less than desirable." This is something we've all been guilty of. Here's how to bring that habit to a halt:

Find something you like about the way you look. Recognize and appreciate it as an admirable quality. Then something else and something else. Completely ignore everything you decided in the past was "not right about the way you look," everything from extra weight to that nose that is too big, to bunions, to the awful __ and the terrible __ and the disgusting __ " ... *Enough,* already!

Instead, shift your attention to what you *do* like: "I like my hands," "I have pretty eyes," "I have nice teeth," "I know I have a cute smile," "I like the dimple on my cheek," "I've always admired my freckles." Go ahead, admit you like those qualities. There's no need to be humble.

Continue that process until you can feel some genuine liking for your physical appearance. Continue some more. Keep doing it until you're not thinking about the way you look. That doesn't mean you don't apply the procedures in this book. It means you apply them as a natural course of action, with your attention extroverted, not introverted.

Now that you've found some physical qualities you genuinely appreciate, let's take a look at how you can further enhance your self-confidence. Here's how:

Let your outer beauty be a reflection of your natural inner beauty. How do you find your inner beauty? Find something you truly like about yourself: The way you walk, the way you hold your spoon, the way you hum a tune. Anything. Then another thing. Then another. Then another. Those qualities are emanating from within you.

Ignore all the "buts": "But I'm not smart like my sister," "I don't know how to dance," etc., etc. Ignore that. Put your attention on what you do like (you can *always* find something!) and keep doing that.

Persist in finding your unique physical qualities, natural abilities and ways you express yourself, those you appreciate, those you like even if it's just a little, and those you love: "I laugh easily," "I'm good at math," "I love to sew," etc., etc., etc. There's *a lot*!

As you continue, you'll discover it's natural. It's not "work." Let yourself shine, bit by bit until the essence of you starts to manifest. Before you know it, your confidence will start to soar and that nasty self-criticism will reduce to a minimum or take a hike completely.

What a great day that is! You're home. You've built your foundation of self-love and self-respect. From that day forward; day by day, week by week, year by year you will be astounded at the amount of your unique qualities and innate abilities that continue to manifest. All because you built that foundation of self-respect.

In the process of strengthening what's right, you may just find that you don't care about bunions or that extra twenty pounds anymore. The weight can fall off naturally because you now see how absolutely fabulous you are no matter what.

There is nothing more beautiful than a woman at peace with herself. When she loves herself she doesn't care how others view her or her looks. But she's beautiful. Isn't that interesting? It's something to recognize.

If you're thinking to yourself, "If beauty is just an attitude, then why did I buy this book?" know that you need to apply the mechanics: the tried-and-true procedures that work as outlined earlier. You can spend your entire life (and definitely get results) caring for the body and how it looks, but if you want to go the whole way it's vital to understand all aspects of the subject we're now addressing. It all works together, your body, your mind and you, the spiritual being.

When you feel good about yourself, you're able to make a stand in other areas of your life. You're not thrown off easily.

The richness of a woman's physical and spiritual beauty comes to full expression through loving herself and living by her true values without compromise. There's nothing more beautiful than a woman who treasures herself for who she is.

> *I do believe that the single most important thing I could ever share with you with regard to maximizing the health, harmony, and happiness in your life can be summed up in just two words: "Love Yourself"*
>
> **Mike Dooley, inspirational author**

Chapter Sixteen

"Aging": Real or Not Real?

et's take up that disagreeable subject of "aging." Why is *even the idea* of aging stressful? It's taken "for granted." It implies a whole catalogue of "inevitabilities," something that is "pre-determined by some unseen force or some decision maker." It tells you there's no choice.

Well, guess what? You can change that. The *real* decision maker is you. It's your choice whether you want to agree or disagree with that subtle or obvious group idea of what "is."

Disagree. It's okay. You'll feel a whole lot better. You may say, "Excuse me? Just how do I do that?" Don't despair. We'll get to that.

In China, the Hunza people live to over one hundred years of age. The women have babies up to age eighty. The men are not well-respected until they get to over a hundred. They are vibrant and alive. We could assume that's true only because of their diet, stress-free environment and overall healthy life-style.

But let's look at something. They are secluded away from all other societies. They don't know that almost everyone else on the planet lives to seventy or eighty years old. They're not indoctrinated in believing in any other way than what they live every day. They agree among themselves they will live happy, healthy lives to over one hundred years of age. And they don't need to talk about it. It just is. It's reality.

If you're in your 40s, 50s or 60s and look around and see others of the same or similar age, with their illnesses and wrinkles, it's easy to think "I must be old" or "I must be getting old."

If you have the mindset "I'm old" you may:

  a. Be limiting yourself as to what you can get done and,
  b. in agreeing with "the aging process," before you know it, it happens. You're "old."

You say, "But what about all those aches, pains and wrinkles I have? Doesn't that *prove* I'm old?" No, it doesn't. You just haven't listened to what Mother Nature has been trying to tell you all along. It's a trap. You'll spend your life worrying. Why bother? Disagree and that alone will make you feel better.

What does it matter how many times your body has been around the sun? You're as young as you feel. If you feel 24 or 45, then that's how "old" you are.

Or you can look at it this way, whichever is most real to you. The number (how old your body is) is what it is, but remember, *it's just a number.* And sometimes fifty (or whatever the "age") can be a fabulous number as in fifty pairs of shoes or fifty million dollars, right?

However you want to look at it is okay. I prefer being 24. Twenty-four million dollars works, too. In other words, there's the calendar age and then there's the real age. 24.

It's pretty hard to change the reality of the society in which we live when it's so broadly accepted and *convincing.* My intention here is to point out that it's only agreement that keeps things "as they are." We don't want to feel like we're the only one, so it's easy to gravitate towards others of like mind and problems.

The process of agreement is inconspicuous and harmful. It slides in unknowingly and becomes a part of you. The more inconspicuous it is, the more harmful. Then it becomes a life-style. And before you know it, you're old and you have lots of friends who have agreed to aches, pains and aging, too.

Now if you're in your 20s or 30s and others warn you of future aching bones, etc., etc., and if you say to yourself, "They must be right because that's the way it is," then you're buying into it and the future can look pretty grim. Horrible thought. There's absolutely no rational reason to put yourself through that. Where cultures and peoples are not so indoctrinated and live healthy lives, they stay young, no matter their "age."

In this country there is an obsession with aging. Why? Because we've agreed to it and have messed with Mother Nature. And we forgot how this whole "aging" thing came about. We're trapped in an agreed-upon body mentality that inhibits one from living life fully as spiritual beings. So guess what? The cosmetic industry and plastic surgeons are making a fortune.

It's a trap. You can never win at it. It's not the real game. The real game is living life the way you want to live it, implementing the basics with your body and feeling great which allows your own fabulous and unique light to shine through.

If we're ever going to live, really live, then we have to recognize the "whim of fate" is a lie. You can apply what you learn in this book and still feel old if you agree with it.

When you talk to people who look and feel half their age, what else are they doing besides taking good care of themselves? They *decided* to be young, feel good and look good. A decision is something you choose of your own free will in spite of anything. That decision is a powerful one.

Know what you want with clarity. When you clearly identify it for yourself, it will happen. The concept applies to any area of one's life. Decide, get very specific and the rest will follow...

Decisions...

Let me tell you a story about my father to exemplify the power of decision.

Many years ago I went home to Colorado to visit. It was six months before his 70th birthday. He was tall and proud and his hair was mostly black with some silver framing his face. He didn't look like the average 69 year-old man. During that same visit he told me he knew he would be "old" when he got to 70.

Six months later I came back for his 70th birthday party. He had slumped at least three inches in height and his hair was solid white. He looked old. The decision that he would be old when he hit 70 came true.

He made it come true through his decision. And it manifested in the way his body changed, *in six months!*

Science can't explain why an 80 year-old woman can lift a car off a child trapped under it. It's because she decided to. Science says she did it because she got a rush of adrenaline. Of course she did. But she had to decide first and then her body cooperated.

There's always a decision first; good or bad. It's our own choice. When a powerful decision is made, heaven and earth move.

I'm sure you've heard a million times that we get what we put our attention on. That is one of the most powerful, basic truths in this or any universe. We make happen what we decide. You've probably heard the saying "energy follows thought." Isn't that true with everything? We don't get going with anything we do in life unless we decide first.

We decide to go to the grocery store, we decide to get a new job, we decide to make a change of some kind. And then we do it. Why can't we also decide for ourselves regarding "aging"? It's the same. Just decide and live it. Don't think about it. Just do it. Ignore all those silly thoughts that you "can't," no matter how *absolutely convincing they are*. If you allow yourself to operate off those "can't" thoughts, you will lose. Guaranteed.

Here's an interesting test you might try sometime that shows just how powerful thoughts can be. With one arm outstretched to the side, have a friend put their palm on the top of your wrist. Then think to yourself "yes, yes, yes," with a full positive feeling and attitude. Don't think about anything, just the "yes!" happily. Have your friend push down on your wrist with their palm. If you were truly positive, your arm will get stronger.

Now do the same thing thinking "no, no, no," while feeling negatively. When your friend pushes down on your wrist you'll see that your arm has gone weak.

This test brings to life how our thoughts strengthen or weaken us and our bodies.

Who's Really Running the Show?

You.

The majority of the world's populations know they are spiritual beings and not their body, with certainty. They don't question it. To them, the idea that we live only one life would be as unnatural to them as saying there is no air to breathe or no sun to come up every day.

The subject can be very confusing. We commonly hear ourselves and others saying "my soul," "my spirit," as a possession. It's not a possession. It's you. You don't own a spirit or soul. You're it.

In the book *The Philosophy of Chiropractic,* B. J. Palmer, the Developer of Chiropractic, says: *"Innate Intelligence is the term applied to the life within the body. We might say it is that which constitutes 'You.'"*

He also says: *"Innate is self-existent, remains unchanged, is not a part of mental or physical manifestation; but instead controls these . . ."*

Note how one naturally says, "My leg," "My hand," etc. One's body is a possession. It doesn't own us. We own it.

One's body responds to the life force controlling it. That life force is you. You're a spiritual being with unlimited potential. You can decide anything.

You can decide you're 24 or whatever age you want to be. I do every day. I don't tell anyone because if I did I would get all sorts of reactions, as in rolling eyes as if to say, "She's having a fun time fooling herself, isn't she?"

But if you really decided you're 24, you'd have another whole life in front of you, right? Now, be 24. There's nothing to lose, just a new perspective to gain; one that sheds light on possibilities and opportunities that seemingly weren't there before.

One's body responds to the life force controlling it. You.

> *Each of us is here to discover our real self... that essentially we are spiritual beings who have taken manifestation in physical form... that we're not human beings that have occasional spiritual experiences... that we're spiritual beings that have occasional human experiences."*
>
> **Deepak Chopra**

The Quality Known as Ageless

In the late 60's I lived in Aspen, Colorado. I have a dear friend there whose name is Peter. Back then I couldn't even begin to estimate his age. I thought it was anywhere from 25 to 35, at the most.

A few years ago I went back to Aspen and visited him. He still has smooth skin and a twinkle in his eye. I asked him how "old" he is. He said 94. I did the math. If he was 94, how old was he back in the 60s? Let's see .... What? He was 57 years old!

Peter seems to live outside time and space. He is wise and kind. The thing that stands out about Peter is that he has never tried to live up to anyone else's expectations of him. He never agreed. He found his own peace. He is ageless.

Do you think the stresses and strains of trying to fit in or look good could bring about aging all by itself? Look at that. Is that possible? Stress due to obsession with aging will alone give a population wrinkles from frown lines!

It's all about:

1. Recognizing your own spirituality and,
2. living the life you want to live, not a life dictated by "shoulds"— yours or others.

It can be difficult for a person to change their mind about something or be receptive to new information unless the old is looked at, inspected for its true value and any falsehoods discarded. We compare ourselves to others and think that's how we should think, act and look because "that's the way it is."

I cannot speak for anyone what falsehoods have been imparted or agreed upon. All I can do is do my best to shed some truth so you can disagree according to your own choice.

Look at the things that have been said to you about aging and the thoughts you've had about it. Then disagree. It's magic. It works. Just keep doing it and you'll be free of the "agreement" even if you have an ache or pain or two or some wrinkles. Keep seeing yourself as young and beautiful, every day, *no matter what*!

One witnesses agelessness in those who know they are spiritual beings.

Nutrition for the Soul

Anti-aging has become an enormous subject of interest. We want to live long, fulfilling, healthy lives and anything that is a threat to that is considered our enemy.

Here's another aspect to anti-aging:

What does your sense of your spirituality, the essence of You, have to do with anti-aging? Much has been said about these two subjects and their relationship to each other, but not enough.

We have bodies with certain nutritional requirements. If those requirements are not met on a daily basis, the effects of physical aging are felt. In the same way, we as spiritual beings have certain daily requirements and if they are not met, we suffer, and we can "age."

Each one of us has needs that we hold dear, needs that give our life meaning when fulfilled. These needs are nutrition for the soul.

I think we can all agree that love is at the top of the list of basic needs. Love is like the air. It's essential. With air and love, we can breathe freely. Giving and receiving love puts everything else into balance and life is much, much simpler, more beautiful and fulfilling. There is nothing that cannot be healed with love, with compassion, with understanding and with laughter.

Each person has their own intimate concept of what "nutrition for the soul" is to them. If you take a look at what that is for you, you can see what makes you whole. My friend Debbie came up with a new term: "Soul Investment."

Invest in those things that complete you.

When you do that "time" is then not a relentless march. Time disappears and life becomes whole.

Chapter Seventeen

Relationships

The People in Your Life:
the Magnificent, the Fallen Angels
and the Darth Vaders!

*W*ow!
The friends in our lives!
How important are they?

The quality of your friendships *can make or break you*. That's a strong statement, I know. But it's true. Please let me repeat that: *The quality of your friendships can make or break you.*

As we just went over, stress is a key factor in aging, health and beauty, if not the number one factor. Because of that, I've taken the liberty of including an aspect of our lives that plays such an important part in our well-being, or lack of.

The friends in our lives can create joy for us or they can create stress for us. It can be hard to accept that certain friends can make our lives tough or tougher.

Nurturing relationships are a buffer against stress and help keep us mentally and physically healthy. We all need people in our lives we can openly talk to without being judged or criticized. When we have true friends, weathering the storms of life is much, much easier.

Many years ago I was going through a period where I felt I wasn't growing in my friendships. Not only that, I was putting so much energy into them and receiving nothing back that I was starting to feel drained. It was making it very difficult to achieve my dreams. It was stressful.

I had two dear friends who lived in another state, but I needed friends close by, friends who could exchange the kind of life-nurturing needs we all have.

We all know it's better to give than receive. But there comes many a time when one's life force has to be replenished so we can *continue* helping. When the "cup is empty," there's nothing more to give, then one feels the need to retreat and recharge. And oftentimes one can feel resentful.

How many times have you thought or heard someone say, "Look at all I've done for ____(name of a person)"? When I have that thought, I know I've chosen the wrong friend to give my unconditional help to. That thought won't occur to you when you have the right inner circle of friends. True friends have an innate sense of exchange.

We've all heard the saying "Love is blind." Love can also be blind in friendships just like marriage. But isn't a real friendship like a marriage also...for better, for worse, in sickness and in health...?

The right friends are observant of you. They see when you are in need of something. They ask. And they provide. And you do the same for them because you want to, because it's a joy.

The most important question to ask of any friendship is: *"Are you both doing better in your lives as a result of the connection?"*

What I did many years ago helped me make the clear distinction between types of friends. It was a clinical process, *but it has made all the difference in the quality of my entire life.*

I made five categories of friends. The first category consisted of those friends who I considered family; the Magnificent, my inner circle. I wrote down all the questions I needed to ask myself to clearly determine a Magnificent friend, for me. My dear, Magnificent friend Jim helped me with these.

You may have your own questions, but I hope these are useful to you in getting started. They are:

 ❧ The first two questions are: How do I feel around them?, Do
    I feel better, worse or the same after I've spoken with them?

- ❧ Could we be roommates?
- ❧ Of my girlfriends, can I call them "sister" and of my male friends, can I call them "brother"?
- ❧ Can I say anything to them and not be judged?
- ❧ Can I fully express my opinions on any subject to them?
- ❧ Are they predictable and stable?
- ❧ If and when I'm vulnerable, are they kind, respectful and unconditionally supportive?
- ❧ Are they genuinely interested in me and my well-being?
- ❧ Do they love and admire me openly of their own free will?
- ❧ Do they help me find and achieve my purposes in life?
- ❧ Do they help me extend my reach in the direction of my choice?
- ❧ If they see I'm doing something damaging to myself or others, do they point it out in a way I don't feel criticized?
- ❧ Do they enforce their reality on me or do they gently seek to bring understanding through consulting my reality?
- ❧ Do they help me look at what I can do to handle situations from my own viewpoint?
- ❧ If there's an upset between us, how long does it take to resolve? (For me, fifteen minutes maximum.)
- ❧ Do they hold a grudge or immediately take full responsibility for any part they played in causing the upset themselves?

After looking at the list of questions, I did some soul-searching to discover for myself whether I can also provide the same to my friends. I have consciously and consistently worked on what I was weak on, to where I can now provide them all. After all, that's what I want in my friends. I need to be able to give them the same.

QUALITIES

"Magnificent" means stellar, qualities above the "norm"; those qualities very easy to see because they stand out!

Now, write out the qualities you need and want in friends, those that shine. Things like: helpful, nurturing, courageous, funny, high integrity, competent, kind, etc. Get *very clear* on those qualities in your own words.

Describe them to yourself. You can always add to them while learning from the inevitable experiences we all have—good, bad and indifferent.

Happiness in your friendships is all up to you through choosing the *right* friends. And happiness in your life, to a very large degree, *depends* on the right friends! You can do something about it by being uncompromising in your choices through knowing the qualities in others that best suit you. Then…?

I went through my address book. I categorized. I wrote down the names of every friend who was Magnificent. There weren't many, in fact painfully few. But at least I was clear in what I needed in a friend.

After I did that, lo and behold, one by one, they started showing up in my life. I am now blessed with several in my inner circle, friends who are true treasures, ones I can call "soul mates." I feel so lucky. But "luck" isn't what did it. It started with clearly defining what I needed in my friendships.

The next category I looked at was friends who fulfilled every need except one: I couldn't say just anything to them. That's okay. They're still dear friends. Knowing there are friends who I don't feel comfortable saying anything to has helped me a lot. I became clear on what subjects can't be talked about with each one of them by knowing what problems between us are not able to get resolved in fifteen minutes or less. I know where to draw the line so either one or both didn't get upset or stay upset. And I can love them even more.

The next category is:

THE FALLEN ANGELS

These are friends who can't reciprocate now. They've "fallen" or they're wounded. They're vulnerable. But they're good people and deserve help. I'm sure you've had fallen angels in your life. We all do at some time or another.

Have you ever heard of "The Goose" story? It beautifully portrays the answer to the question of "What do you do with Fallen Angels?"

Here it is:

Next fall, when you see geese heading South for the winter, flying along in a "V" formation, you might consider what science has discovered as to why they fly that way. As each bird flaps its wings, it creates uplift for the bird immediately following. By flying in "V" formation the whole flock adds at least 71% greater flying range than if each bird flew on its own.

People who share a common direction and sense of community can get where they are going more quickly and easily because they are traveling on the thrust of one another.

When a goose falls out of formation it suddenly feels the drag and resistance of trying to go it alone and quickly gets back into formation to take advantage of the lifting power of the bird in front.

If we have as much sense as a goose, we will stay in formation with those who are headed in the same way we are. When the head goose gets tired it rotates back in the wing and another goose flies the point.

It is sensible to take turns doing demanding jobs with other people or with geese flying South. Geese honk from behind to encourage those up front to keep up their speed. What do we say when we honk from behind?

Finally—and this is important—when a goose gets sick and falls out of formation, two other geese fall out with that goose and follow it down to lend help and protection. They stay with the fallen goose until it is able to fly, and only then do they launch out on their own, or with another formation, to catch up with their group.

If we have the sense of a goose we will stand by each other like that.

Author Unknown

That pretty much says it all about these valuable, but temporarily broken friends, doesn't it? Help them and don't expect anything back until they are once again head of the flock and can carry you on the wind of their wings.

The next category is those who are Acquaintances. These are people you have met and like but don't know well. They may eventually move into the category of Magnificent!

THE DARTH VADERS

Now, the one you can't wait to hear about. We all know about the villain "Darth Vader" as Anakin Skywalker in Star Wars, a symbol of evil.

He vowed he would get his mother out of slavery. When he failed, he went crazy and wiped out the village where she was enslaved. The loss of his mother was so great that when the Dark Chancellor approached

Anakin and told him if he went to the Dark Side, he could learn how to bring someone back to life. Anakin couldn't resist.

Anakin tried to turn his son Luke over to the Dark Side also. We know that in the end Luke succeeds in bringing his father back to the good side of the Force.

So, why am I bringing this up?

I have three "Darths" in my past. Each turned to the Dark Side in an effort to solve a problem, the same as Darth Vader.

I was blinded by my love for them. I tried converting them back, but it took an enormous amount of time and energy I could no longer expend. Someday, they will return to the good side. I have forgiven them, but I keep them at arm's length.

I leave the decisions to you on how to handle "the dark ones" in your life.

It's *very helpful* to write down the names of those people who fall into each of the categories: The Magnificent, ones with a "taboo" subject, fallen angels, acquaintances and Darth Vaders.

Most importantly, know that calling the Magnificent Ones into your life will bring you joy. Joy is the opposite of stress. At times my friends can be grouchy and volatile. No one's perfect. But their strengths satisfy my needs and my strengths satisfy theirs. I can live with imperfections, including mine.

> "... let there be no purpose in friendship save the deepening of the spirit."
>
> **Kahlil Gibran**

What about the Other People in Our Lives?

We all have bosses, people we have to answer to, co-workers, acquaintances. What if any of these relationships are less than ideal?

Here's an awakening statement: Stress due to anyone in our lives making us feel small, inadequate or uncertain in reaching towards our goals is a key factor in illness. Unfortunate, but true.

What does one do when the atmosphere around certain people is consistently less than pleasant, when every time you see them you get a knot in your stomach? You have to be the judge of what you want to do about it. But maybe this will help.

The questions still apply: "How do I feel around them?" "Do I feel better, worse or the same after I've spoken with them?" But if they're having a bad day or going through a particularly stressful time themselves, don't judge them. We all have bad days and tough times. It's how you feel around them consistently, good or bad, over the long term that counts.

Remember, the majority of difficulties with others stem from lack of communication. There may be a misunderstanding between you. Work it out. Talk it all the way through. Take responsibility yourself. In the process, you may have some "Aha!" moments—moments when you discover there was a misunderstanding. Who knows? Find out. And this doesn't mean texting or emailing back and forth. It's face-to-face or over the phone when you can't meet in person.

Remember it's not what is said, it's how it's said. Communication coming from care is always well-received.

If you find that person just isn't receptive and even if they are but the problem between you still doesn't resolve, then you have to look at where you want to draw the line. If the relationship is very important to you, it takes more energy, energy equal to how valuable it is to you.

All relationships are an investment of time and energy. You have to evaluate its worth. Decide where you want to put that time and energy and act accordingly. If you can't get anywhere, it needs to be recognized as such.

Decide on the kind of people you want in your life and seek them out. Keep your life force shining through having nurturing relationships and assist others to do the same. *Your happiness and their happiness depend on it.*

Now, what about those who make a practice of introverting others?

The fortunate part is, there aren't many.

You've just returned from the hairdresser over lunch. Your hair looks like it was just put through a meat grinder. To top it off, it's orange. You *can't wait* to get to the ladies room to try to put some order into the tangled mess and wash out the color. Before you land at the ladies room door, a co-worker, in front of everyone, yells out "Susie! You look *sooooooo* good today! Who does your hair?" He laughs, but it's not funny. It's the same guy who will poke at your stomach and say, "Put on a little weight, Susie?"

An extremely helpful guide that can help in these situations is the Credo of Mother Teresa:

"People are often unreasonable, irrational, and self centered; Forgive them anyway. If you are kind, people may accuse you of selfish, ulterior motives; Be kind anyway. If you are successful, you will win some unfaithful friends and some genuine enemies; Succeed anyway. If you are honest and sincere people may deceive you; Be honest and sincere anyway. What you spend years creating others could destroy overnight; Create anyway. If you find serenity and happiness, some may be jealous; Be happy anyway. The good you do today will often be forgotten; Do good anyway. Give the best you have, and it may never be enough; Give your best anyway. In the final analysis it is between you and God, It was never between you and them anyway."

That's certainly the ideal to strive for, isn't it?

How do we put this to practical use in the everyday world? There's nothing wrong and everything right with kindly saying to your co-worker, while looking at him straight in the eye, "I don't like what you're doing. Stop," or whatever is appropriate depending on the circumstance. He may defend himself, justify his behavior by saying "I'm just teasing you. Don't be so sensitive," try to insult you further, go off in a huff, or anything else. By letting him calmly, but firmly, know you're aware of what he's doing, you're doing your part in protecting yourself and others from being treated badly. It's a guarantee that same coworker is treating others with disrespect, too.

We can't continue to allow a small percentage of people make ourselves or others feel small.

Forgive that person but don't let them shake your certainty of who you are and the values you stand for.

In applying this, before you know it the other people in the office will listen to you. When you have certainty of your own viewpoint, you don't care what others think of you. Say what's on your mind. Those of kindred spirit will think you're awesome. They're your friends.

The key here is knowing, protecting and nurturing your own ideas about yourself and about life. "Fitting in" or being smaller just to be part of the group is a trap. Do you want to be like everyone else? I hope not because there's no one in the world like you. No one.

How to Win a Man's Heart

I can't resist. You want to know how to win a man's heart? It's simple. So simple it hurts.

It's not by having silicone breasts and collagen lips but by being yourself and letting your own natural beauty shine through. Yes, that's right. You don't want the kind of man who will marry you for your breasts. He'll leave you for the next pair that comes along.

Some men like big breasts, some like shapely legs, and some like beautiful eyes or a size 2. Are you going to spend your life trying to fit that picture? Or are you going to validate your natural assets, let them truly shine and win the man of your dreams; the one who loves you for your beautiful shining, unique self?

It's pretty clear which relationship is going to be fulfilling and last for a lifetime.

YOUR MAN

Since we're on the subject of men, what about how they feel?

Let's not fool ourselves. We women, along with wanting to look and feel beautiful for ourselves, want to look and feel beautiful for the male gender. If we didn't, we wouldn't bother with everything we do to be attractive. And the multi-million dollar beauty-care industry wouldn't exist.

When you're happy through taking good care of yourself, your man knows he's important to you because you're also making that special effort to be happy for him too.

No matter what, men need our natural radiance and inspiration in their lives. It's very challenging indeed to be our naturally radiant selves or an inspiration to anyone if we're not rested and doing what we need to do for ourselves to be happy and fulfilled.

Depending on your circumstances, whether you're a single, working mom or married to a man of means and don't have to bring in income, there's still a responsibility in taking care of yourself.

If you don't have a man in your life right now, looking and feeling the way you want to feel and look will open the door to the *right* man finding you, as you.

WHEN YOU'RE HAPPY, HE'S HAPPY

There's an old saying, *"When the woman is happy, the man is happy."* It starts with you and having the courage to ask for his support in giving you the space and time and yes, if needed, financial help to be delicious and happy.

In this day and age the reality of a woman being a stay-at-home mom and not employed may have questions as to its workability, but you can always work it out as long as it makes good sense to both of you and it's what you both want.

I remember the wife of a client who sat in front of me sobbing because her husband wanted her to work with him in his business. She wanted to stay home and be a full-time mom. That's what would make her happy. Little did he know how *his* future depended on her following her heart.

Don't keep longing to do what's natural to you. Take charge. The rest will follow.

If you're a single, working mom you have a different challenge. If you have decided to never have another thing to do with a man, if I may be so bold, I don't believe you. Underneath that hurt is a woman who longs to be loved and to love. And there are men out there longing to love and be loved too. Find him or let him find you.

There's also the saying, *"Behind every successful man is a good woman."* That's the woman who fulfills her role as a woman *because she wants to.* That doesn't mean you don't work. That means you account for everything else too: your health, your rest, your beauty, your happiness and work out how that can realistically be done, with your man.

Understand no one, least of all me, is suggesting putting you in a box: matter of fact, just the opposite. The question is: *Where do you feel your life force flowing effortlessly?* For me, my "job" is not work, but I work hard and love what I do. It's all about being honest with yourself about what fulfills you and makes you whole. A woman anchored in her own integrity and radiance can live her true nature and naturally benefit everyone around her by being herself.

The fact remains that men and women are different. Each should hold to their basic nature and value the best in each other and what the other has to offer. Creating agreement and power between a man and a woman allows both to fulfill what is meaningful for them individually and together as a team.

I remember a fitting excerpt from a book called *The Popcorn Report* by Faith Popcorn. She predicts trends in the marketplace. She sees that women are the vanguards of the future, now more than ever. The materialism in the world needs to be balanced out with the spiritual side; the side a woman brings. A woman is the living work of art that raises the quality of life for everyone.

Get very clear and specific on the changes you wish to make in your life; how you're going to begin taking care of yourself physically and spiritually and continue doing so. Then let your man know what the changes are, one at a time. Prepare him for the new you, and let him gradually get used to it. Everyone will win, including him. He'll value seeing you take charge in your rightful role as a woman.

Here is a quote by a man who recognized and treasured the value of women:

> *"Whenever women have insisted on absolute equality with men, they have invariably wound up with the dirty end of the stick. What they are and what they can do makes them superior to men, and their proper tactic is to demand special privileges, all the traffic will bear. They should never settle merely for equality. For women, 'equality' is a disaster."*
> **Robert A. Heinlein**
> **from the book "Time Enough for Love"**

Chapter Eighteen

How Do I Achieve Happiness?

My goodness. How do we create that? Have you heard the lyrics to the song by Carol King?—"You've got to wake up every morning with a smile on your face and show the world all the love in your heart."?

Many days I sing and dance all by myself while I'm doing household chores. It doesn't matter if I sing off key or act like I'm two years old. I have a great time entertaining myself because I'm not trying to impress anyone. My man comes home and with a silly grin on my face, I smother him with kisses or continue the playfulness. I'm not happy only because he loves me. I've created my own happiness. It works out that way.

You know the saying "girls just want to have fun"? Well, it's true. We do. We're here to lighten the load with our girlishness. And a man loves to see his woman with a smile on her face.

Many years ago, I lived with a friend in the lower part of her house on the water. We called it "The Veranda Room." Each morning upon awakening I would sit out on my front patio and watch the birds: the pelicans performing their vertical dives, the big grey heron commanding the water around him, the soaring seagulls with their unmistakable squawking. Then one morning I saw a smaller bird I couldn't name, but he stood out above all the others. He was splashing in the water, as cute and silly as could be. He was trying to tell those other birds, so intent on survival, "Isn't this fun, isn't this grand? Here we are, we have this playground all around us! Look at these great waves! Come on, let's play!"

One bird, all by himself, the natural comedian of the bay, looking for playmates.

Later that afternoon I came outside and saw him maneuvering his way up the steps alongside my porch. As he bounced from step to step, he casually looked at me as if to say, "Don't bother me. I'm exploring. Hey! What's upstairs?"

Remember the book Jonathan Livingston Seagull, the seagull that ventured out on his own, hungry and tired, to see how high he could soar? Well, this cute, silly bird's mission in life was to play, to have adventure, to discover the magic. And that's what he did.

You may ask, how does one play, find adventure and magic in every day? Sometimes in life, it can seem difficult to find things to be interested in. You may say, "I need lots of money to do those things."

A few years back I was really bored. (There's nothing worse!) Then a long-time friend asked me to go for a walk. As we were walking and talking, he stopped and picked up a pecan under a tree. While continuing our walk, I noticed he was squeezing and rubbing the pecan in his hand. Without missing a beat, he took my hand, placed the pecan in my palm, wrapped my fingers around it and held my hand tight in his. We continued the same conversation we had started, yet another "conversation" was happening: one that was having a profound impact on me.

I wanted to experience what he had by holding and rolling that pecan in his palm with such fascination. He let go of my hand. I knew he wanted me to feel what he felt; the texture, the life that pulsed in it, the rawness of it, the sublime beauty of simplicity. I did.

We held a timeless space of understanding without uttering a word about it. I felt re-born with a new perspective on life. That's all it took.

It has been my purpose all along to fill the spaces with magic. It's my bliss. In the course of life you'll find your bliss and your joy if you let it happen. It's these moments; the new, fun, innocent and enlightening experiences, the ones that allow in the real messages we seek; food for the soul. Surrender to them.

A dear friend of mine has a wonderful quote: *"One should live in awe of one's own existence."*

It would be therapeutic to sit down and write down those moments of awe you've had by yourself and with others. It would accomplish two things; it would give you a reminder of what brings you personal joy and second, if you sent it to your friends, it would remind them of the joy you've shared together and what's magical in life.

> *"Life is not the amount of breaths you take. It's the moments*
> *that take your breath away."*
> **From the movie Hitch – Kevin Bisch, screenwriter**

HUMOR

Do you remember a time someone said something so funny, you were taken completely off guard and laughed until you had tears rolling uncontrollably down your cheeks?

Silly attacks. What's that? That's being absolutely goofy, where you laugh so hard, that everything "serious" is well... just silly.

Several years ago a good friend of mine, a very proper English gentleman, took me to breakfast. For starters he ordered half a grapefruit. As I'm watching him cut each little wedge of grapefruit in painstaking detail, place each bite in his mouth with perfect precision and manners while sitting fully upright in the booth, I'm bursting with suppressed laughter. Mind you, I have nothing against perfect manners. Matter of fact, just the opposite. But this seemed just a bit over the top for an American cowgirl.

As he notices the orange juice I just took a swallow of is about to come out through my nose while I'm doing everything I can to smother the outburst of laughter just below the surface, he calmly places his grapefruit knife and fork down on the table, and without missing a beat or changing the prim expression on his face, scoops up the half grapefruit with both palms and proceeds to "juice" it on his face. I mean, really juice it, back and forth until the juice is dripping down his face and the pulp hanging from his cheeks. I lost it. My suppressed glee erupted and no one in the restaurant saw what was so funny which of course made it even funnier.

Silly attacks—the best!

My friend Jack has a saying: "We have two choices: one is to laugh and the other is to cry. I choose to laugh." He maintains a sense of humor throughout every trial he faces. He always finds the light and humorous side of any situation, watches comedy, tells a funny story or joke or makes a silly face.

It's hard to remain serious in the face of lightheartedness.

What, my friends, makes one person feel younger and happier than another? Here's the answer:

> "The reason angels can fly is that they take themselves lightly."
> **G.K. Chesterton**

And another...

> "We don't stop playing because we grow old; we grow old because we stop playing."
> **George Bernard Shaw**

Be good to yourself, laugh and have fun!

Find Your Joys

Would you like to wake up in the morning, excited to get going with the day; where you can't wait to _____? It doesn't matter what it is. Even if you're going to your regular job, there's always something to be excited about, some delightful experience awaiting you.

It's what fills your cup to overflowing! When your cup is filled to overflowing, it starts to splash over into other people's lives and the other aspects of living. That's when opportunities start to open up. That's when "serendipity" happens! ("Serendipity" means wonderful surprising things happening "by chance.")

Remember Rivka, the one who woke me up to my purpose as a woman? One morning I arrived in her kitchen to behold her in a dance; a graceful, playful and delightful flow to an Israeli song, swirling a spoon around in the air in tune with the music while alternately stirring the soup she had just made, dressed in her beautiful, colorful clothes with a flower in her hair and singing.

Later that morning she stuck her face in a honey jar like Pooh (from Winnie the Pooh), then looked sideways at me with such innocence on her face that I melted. You had to be there. You would have melted too.

> *"Step number one for changing the entire world, is falling in love*
> *with it as it already is. The same is true for changing yourself."*
> **Mike Dooley, Author**

DOING WHAT'S IMPORTANT TO YOU

> *"A man (person) is a success if he gets up in the morning and*
> *goes to bed at night and in between does what he wants to do."*
> **Bob Dylan**

I'm conveying this information to you because it directly relates to whether a person is happy in life or not. When a person is happy, there's much less stress, or stress becomes non-existent. Let's take a brief look at something important.

How many people do you know who are really, genuinely happy? Not many, huh? Most people are living off "shoulds." How dreary.

Of the hundreds of people I've worked with, I've found very few on their own paths. There were always one or more "things" that prevented them from being themselves in life or giving full expression to their personal dreams with no compromise. One for one, they were all making less of their abilities.

Many years ago I asked several women to tell me what they would be doing in life right now if they could. I had the most surprising and interesting reactions from many of them. Terror. Yes, terror. I was quite amazed by this as you can imagine. Then I asked myself why this is and then realized I have also experienced it. Challenge.

Most people are afraid of testing their abilities, testing themselves, "moving out of the box." On and off I've been guilty of not following my dreams until I got disenchanted enough with myself to disagree with barriers; my own and those others put before me. I would find out who my friends really were if I followed my dreams. And in finding out, I now have a circle of best friends, those who encourage and support my endeavors fully. Others fell by the wayside and are still living a life of compromise.

Are you doing what you want to do?

This is not easy to look at. How does not being true to oneself create stress? That's a very interesting question. It's because one is internally fighting one's own personal needs. Don't fight. Just do what's important to you.

Do you remember times when you did something you truly wanted to do, even if it was only for a day and how you felt?

Shopping. We women love to shop. I do. The saying "Shop 'til you drop" says we have that purpose that not even tiredness can get in the way of. Imagine feeling that way most of the time. Not real? Okay. Just try it.

Shopping for shopping's sake will outlive its excitement once we have all the clothes we want. So where do we go from there?

There's nothing more exciting than demonstrating your abilities and being able to say, "I did it!"

When you've accomplished something in life, you utilized one or more of your abilities—abilities you perhaps didn't even know you had until a situation called for one or more of them.

Let me give you an example: You sing in a choir. The lead singer backs out at the last moment before a major performance. You're asked to fill the part. You're anything from surprised to terrified to shocked. Doesn't matter. The show must go on and you've been chosen. You've had no time to prepare. You do it because you have to. You get on stage and even though you may go off key a few times, you sing the best you've ever sung in spite of being nervous or even terrified.

Now other opportunities open up because you didn't lose your nerve. You found you had courage. That's an ability. You found you could hit higher notes than you ever thought. That's an ability. You found you could have the spotlight on you. That's an ability. We *all* have those moments, big, medium or small.

There are abundant abilities inherent in you crying out to be demonstrated.

Write your natural and acquired abilities down. Look at them for what they are. There's no need to be humble. It's the truth, so flaunt them to yourself and continue giving full expression to them in daily living. If you do this, more and more previously unrecognized and un-utilized abilities will surface and will continue to do so as you journey through life. Recognizing and then demonstrating those abilities allows you to discover how truly amazing you are. That's plays *a very key part* in ensuring your happiness. Happiness in life means stress is taking a back seat.

It's interesting to observe that we're the most proud of those accomplishments that have contributed to others: everything from taking that lead in a performance, to helping a friend get past a crisis, to winning a race for your team, to graduating from college, or having a flower garden. You wanted it for yourself, you got it! And the people around you loved it, too. You made a difference in their lives. You gave them license to win for themselves also.

Within *every* person is their own native creativeness. Everyone is an artist. If you say, "But, I'm not an artist!" look again. The expression of your own being placed in the universe is your art.

Everyone has had one or more times in their lives, through the use of their natural and/or acquired abilities and unique personality, whether it lasted for two minutes or two years, times when they shined.

That's art. That's you.

Make sense? I hope so.

Orison Swett Marden, a prolific author of success and motivational books, wrote:

> *"Deep within man dwell those slumbering powers; powers that would astonish him, that he never dreamed of possessing; forces that would revolutionize his life if aroused and put into action."*

Forces that would revolutionize his life if aroused and put into action...

Conquering Your Life

> *"Your ship was spotted off the coast this morning, slipping silently through the fog...coming around the cape she appeared in a shaft of sunlight...and what a sight to see! Glimmering as much as the ocean herself. Massive and*

beautiful beyond belief! Laden with treasures, happy times,
friends, love and laughter. Quick, you must PREPARE
for her docking...you MUST make space in your life for her
gifts...otherwise, just as quickly, she'll quietly slip back out
to sea."

Mike Dooley, Author

How many people do you know never get to what they really want to do
because they're so tied up in the mechanics of daily living?

Probably just about everyone. We all have work and the usual chores
which of course have to get done. But if a person doesn't feel they can
move forward toward their dreams, life becomes "the same ole, same ole."
And that's a sure route to unhappiness. We love to feel inspired and love
the challenges to know we're alive, because we are alive. We might as well
be *really* alive.

PRIORITIES

Most of us know how important it is to prioritize our activities. What
do you consider a priority? What gets you excited to get going with your
day even if you have a regular 9-5 job which most of us do?

I'll let you in on a little secret that has helped me a great deal. Every
morning when I wake up, before getting out of bed, I ask myself "What
activity can I accomplish or what ability can I work on today that gets me
motivated to get going?" I lay for thirty seconds or five minutes or longer
until I find something that inspires me to take action. I always find it. I
always jump out of bed, excited. That's my priority and my duty; to be
excited about life in taking action to make my dreams come true.

Here's another helpful tip: Have a big sign on your wall, right in front
of you where you work most of the time that says: "Is this activity helping
me move forward towards my goal?" If it's not, delay, delegate or dump
it. Put it in your pending basket, out basket or wastebasket. Don't waste
time on actions that won't contribute to your dreams. More practically
speaking, it's called "Time Management."

It's your time. Manage it how you want to.

Create your own system of time management that keeps you excited.

Write out your plan, step-by-step, how you're going to get there. Put your attention on the action steps. Ignore barriers you think might get in your way. Every day re-envision the dream while you're proceeding on the "do" steps one at a time, in sequence.

At one point your dream will take on more and more of a life of its own where soon you can't be stopped. You're building momentum using the speed that works for you.

You'll now find those activities that don't contribute to the materialization of your dreams (like watching TV) will now fall into their proper perspective. They will capture your time and attention less and less and will now be viewed as distractions, to be happily removed.

Every day do a little more of what you want to do and a little less of what you don't. Whittle the mundane activities down to essential ones. In doing this, you will see your dream taking shape in the quote, unquote "real" world. Only this time you're making reality. Your own.

My cousin has a saying: "Plan your work, work your plan." It's not a robotic activity, it's alive and fluid. Be able to switch gears back and forth from obligations to dreams.

Knowing what you want to do and wanting to do it badly enough will get you over the hurdle of doing things that are not exciting for the moment. You know you're getting to what is exciting, today!

> *"Don't let the dazzling heights you aspire to scare you from getting started. After all, few could climb Mt. Everest tomorrow, though virtually all could begin preparing."*
> **Mike Dooley**

INSPIRATION FOR OTHERS

Following your own path is the most unselfish thing you can do. By example, you will dramatically help lift others out of their lives of desperation through letting *your* light shine with no reservations. Others will then know it's possible to be happy by endowing life into *their* dreams.

Have you ever heard or known of people who once struggled and then persisted on their road to personal and/or professional success? As a result they have an abundance of overflowing help to bestow upon others. They made it. Now, they want to help others do the same. That could be you: a Success Story which inspires others to take charge of their own lives.

In your journey you will experience emotions you never thought you had. You will get exhilarated, frustrated, tired, bored, afraid and exhilarated again as you encounter and overcome the barriers. Keep going. Believe me my dear sister, I've experienced everything from the deep emotion of worry to the profound joy of success and everything in-between. I'm no different from you in this way.

The abilities inherent in you are crying out to be demonstrated. You are alive. You are vital. You are amazing and unique. Allow yourself to take big space. Go to a beautiful park, lie on the grass, take a nap and daydream. Just be and let the inspiration come and give thanks when it does.

Have a strong enough purpose to carry you all the way through; the determination to accomplish what's important to you in heart and soul, no matter what. Be bold and daring. Let nothing get in your way.

This is your freedom: living your dreams and helping others do the same. At some point not only will stress start to disappear from your life, but you will be genuinely happy.

> *"The purpose of life is a life of purpose."*
> **Robert Byrnes**

Write down the life you want.
Start to:
see it,
feel it,
hear it,
touch it,
visualize it.
Use your imagination to elaborate on it,
step by step,
making it grow,
while gradually giving it your power.
See each step taking shape.
Now get the idea of living that life,
living it every day,

being more and more empowered by the life force you give it.

You will have it if you do this.

Trust in yourself.

Remember this–it's never too late to get started.

My dear sister, I officially give you permission to do whatever it takes to take not just good, but *great* care of yourself and be happy living the life you want. *Now, give yourself permission.*

Life is an adventure. Live it and bend it to your will.

Gathering the Flame

> *"When you cannot make up your mind which of two evenly balanced courses of action you should take—choose the bolder."*
>
> **W.J. Slim**

I have a confession. You'll see how it all fits.

As a child I had a burning hunger to be on stage. But who did I think I was? I couldn't even raise my hand in a classroom without my heart pounding so hard I thought others could surely hear it. In the spotlight? Forget it!

Twenty-five years later I co-owned a seminar company. My partner was a very powerful and charismatic public speaker and natural comic. He could make the audiences howl with laughter until they rolled in the aisles.

While I sat in the back of the room watching him, I'd think to myself: "I could never do that. I don't have his sense of humor, his charm, his wit, blah, blah, blah." So I gave him center stage and had my own "play" going on quietly (or not so quietly) in the background. I felt a deep loss that I didn't have "what it took." I took my place as the silent, stifled and forlorn partner. But in my heart, I still had a faint remaining hope that maybe, someday, some way I'd conquer my complete horror of standing in front of a group of people and having rotten tomatoes thrown at me. Or much worse; like a guillotine.

For years I couldn't come to terms with myself, to muster up the courage to "speak up!" Then one day, miraculously, out-of-the-blue I woke up. I gave myself a huge, "No more of this pitiful self-denial!" I decided to do *whatever it took* to conquer my stark-raving terror of public speaking.

I didn't talk with anyone about my plan, including my friends. I didn't dare! If I did I'd have to actually prove myself. By now, I think you're getting the idea my fear was *reeeeally* bad.

It all changed with two days of training by a maestro of public speaking.

I managed to make my way to the class, with a raving migraine headache. I made sure no one was there I knew.

To put it mildly his coaching gave me the breakthrough of my life.

In turn, each attendee took their place on stage. The trainer positioned himself at the back of the room listening to each person talk about their favorite animal and where we would like to go on vacation and why. Definite ice-breakers.

Of course, I made sure my turn to speak was at the end of the class. I could then make my fast get-a-way when it was over. But being last turned out to be a real advantage as I had a chance to see what he did with each budding speaker before I made my way to front and center stage.

With each student he ignored everything that was wrong about their presentation and only pointed out what was right, knowing that what we put our attention on gets stronger.

Now, it may sound over-dramatic, in fact everything I've said so far may be sounding over-dramatic, but when I say it was the beginning of a new life, I'm not exaggerating. I saw, before my eyes, every person in the class, including myself, transform from being introverted and shy to confident. And not just confident, but truly shining.

Gone were the days of comparing myself or trying to be like anyone else. I knew my strengths. I ignored the weaknesses. It no longer mattered how dynamic other speakers were. And miracle of all miracles, since then I have spoken to hundreds of people on stage, truly at home in the spotlight, still nervous (as any speaker is when about to go on stage), but at home.

Anyone can overcome their fears and live their dreams. Will it be you? I hope so.

Franklin D. Roosevelt said, *"The only thing we have to fear is fear itself."* That's it, the only thing.

My wish, from the bottom of my heart, is that you've shed some trappings that could restrain you from being and living your magnificent self. Because all that matters is what's right about you.

It is my opinion that maintaining integrity to oneself and following through on one's own goals and purposes in life is the only valid measure of success.

> *"And behold I have found that which is greater than wisdom.*
> *It is a flame spirit in you ever gathering more of itself."*
> **Kahlil Gibran**

"How am I going to change the world?
... or change myself to be a more vital part of it?"

Speak your mind. Speak your heart. Don't be afraid of disagreement or rejection. Bring it on. You know what's true for you. Don't take anyone else's word. Listen only to those who have been successful following their chosen paths, and even then use your own intuitive judgment.

Remember the famous Lewis Carroll quote?

"There is no use trying," said Alice; "one can't believe impossible things."

"I dare say you haven't had much practice," said the Queen.

"When I was your age, I always did it for half an hour a day.

"Why, sometimes I've believed as many as six impossible things before breakfast."

Each one of us has to be able to see ourselves actually living the life we envision. It takes work, sometimes a lot, to bring our ideal about. Persistence in the discovery process is a great challenge you *will* win at if you truly decide.

What you learn along the way is the best part. For me, I never thought I could be a writer until I started writing.

Get help when you need it but only from those who are qualified and have proven success in the area you want to excel in. There are wonderful books available on getting organized to make your dreams happen. And there are also brilliant mentors, coaches and consultants who can help you. Make sure you find one you really click with and will help you with what you want, not what *they* want! Leave the practical aspects to them if you want to. You're the creator of the game.

I hope this section on stress has been enormously useful to you. It's vital we gain control over the factors of stress.

One decision, one action, good or bad, can change the whole direction of your life. Make the positive ones, the ones that lead you to your dreams, ones that will help make this planet a fabulous place to live for you and for those you love.

Gather your flame and let your passion light the world!

> *"The difference between what we do and what we are capable of doing would suffice to solve most of the world's problems."*
> **Mahatma Gandhi**

Conclusion

hy have I taken up the subjects of stress, beauty, your individuality, anti-aging, relationships, fun and following your dreams? What do these ultimately have to do with hair loss and beauty? The contents of this book has been a thorough look at what can ultimately result in hair loss and feeling old; physically, mentally and spiritually. They are all valid, all real.

If these tools seem too simple, remember the only true power there is, is simplicity.

You *can* achieve anything if you demand it. "Wanting" is like the carrot one never reaches. "Demanding" means you won't take no for an answer. If you have one or more strong enough purposes to look, feel and live the way you want, those purposes will carry you through *all* obstacles. It would be silly to imagine not achieving what you want. But if your purposes are not strong enough, those "obstacles" will be enough to throw you off your path.

At that point, rethink your purposes.

Ask yourself any or all of these questions:

- What is it that I *really* want?
- How do I want to look and feel?
- Are those purposes strong enough to carry me all the way through to the result I want?
- Are they really *my* purposes or am I just trying to please others?
- Do I want to look and feel beautiful, for me first?
- Do I need to reword my purposes until that passion is so strong within me that nothing can take me off my chosen path?
- Where will those purposes take me in life?
- Will they help me achieve what I want?

Get *very clear* on them and how they will assist you in all aspects of your life. *After all, it is your life.* Having more than one purpose will, each one, in sequence, further the next and the next...

Be completely honest with yourself. If you want to grow turnips for the next year, do it and don't care what anyone else thinks. You'll find a way to please yourself and everyone else, too.

It's life-changing when one has one or more passionate purposes. Even though it takes a lot of "work," we'll do whatever it takes to make it happen.

One of the reasons for writing this book has been to assist you in stepping out of the box of unworkable ideas we have been so indoctrinated into so we can think for ourselves.

My intention hasn't been to get your attention fixed on your body and how it looks. It's to get you to decide how you want to express yourself. For me, thin hair and "aging" wasn't an option. Thick, beautiful hair, youthful skin and vibrant health was, and still is, an expression of how I want to be viewed; first to myself and then to the rest of the world.

There's no need to treat your body like a temple. It's not. It's here to serve you, not the other way around.

You might be asking yourself: "Will I really apply all these procedures and techniques to change the condition of my hair, scalp and health?" "Is it really worth all this trouble?" If it's not, please don't. I don't want you to do anything against your will. It should be a joy with a distinct goal in mind.

When I asked myself the same question, I had no doubt. The rewards of feeling great most of the time give one a brand-new perspective. Opportunities open up that apparently weren't there before. What is that worth?

If you get too absorbed in the mechanics of looking young and beautiful, then it's easy to forget the reasons for looking and feeling that way in the first place; to feel alive and go forward toward the realization of your dreams with an unstoppable passion. This life is a golden opportunity to experience the happiness you never thought possible. Doors open when you're in high spirits.

It takes a definite personal decision to cause life to work the way we want. No other factor is relevant or gives us more stability than being sure of what we want and going for it.

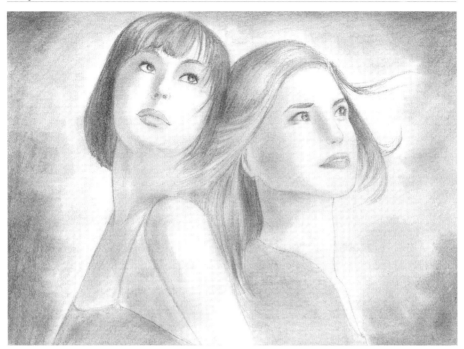

Some of these procedures are going to take more time than others, but with patience and persistence you'll master them. Live and enjoy life as you're implementing them. Concern and worry will add stress and prolong the process. Remember when I mentioned earlier that the first thing I had to do to grow a glorious head of hair was to stop worrying? I decided to have fun in life while watching the hair-repair techniques and health procedures work.

Here's a suggestion to make the implementation process simple: a) find the category of your hair in the charts in the back of the book and, b) highlight those actions you know you can apply right now; those that are easy for you. Once you have mastered those, go on to the next.

Remember, the charts are not a substitute for the full information contained in the body of this book. Referring back to the sections you need in the main text as often as needed will give you certainty.

I incorporated all this into my life gradually. It's now a habit. I am able to feel, look and live the way I want. Having a grand time in life, without the "normal" distractions is wonderful. It's a relief.

We've all experienced information-overload and an endless parade of products that either don't work or harm us in some way. One of my primary intentions in writing this book has been to save you years of trial-and-error and extensive research one experiences in coming up with the simple and workable answers.

I truly hope I've provided you with the answers you've been searching for and much, much more. It's always the basics, the ones that can be applied for an entire life.

"First, when there's nothing but a slow glowing dream
That your fear seems to hide deep inside your mind
All alone I have cried silent tears full of pride
In a world made of steel, made of stone
Well I hear the music, close my eyes, feel the rhythm
Wrap around, take a hold of my heart
What a feeling, bein's believin'
I can have it all, now I'm dancin' for my life
Take your passion, and make it happen
Pictures come alive, you can dance right through your life."
From the movie Flashdance, song written by Irene Cara,
Giorgio Moroder & Keith Forsey

It's Really the Beginning...

Our world and the people occupying it are changing. In my opinion, we have the opportunity now more than ever to make the shift from a mentality governed by materialism to a Renaissance, a rebirth of our spirituality; simply.

There seems to be a more obvious and clear contrast between the forces that would keep us oblivious to the truth and those of truth.

Never has there been such a downward plunge into the possibility of total manipulation by those who would keep man's true spiritual nature clouded, versus an awakening that is happening all over the planet in bringing to light the true virtues and power which reside naturally in each and every one of us.

When we really look at what's happening, we can view those changes and make our own decisions towards the direction we want to go and dedicate ourselves to achieving the end result we want.

More and more people are turning to alternative solutions for their health and well-being instead of depending on others whose interests lie primarily in financial profit through the use of drugs and chemicals.

We can accelerate this alternate process as individuals through seeking those of kindred spirit and endowing those relationships with everything we wish so deeply for ourselves; care.

The beautiful life we wish to live is only possible through our own clear-cut decisions regarding what we value the most; living and standing by it, no matter what.

If we look into the near and distant future and see what we would like it to look like and then ask ourselves "How did we get there?", we'll be telling ourselves the steps we need to take now, in sequence, to arrive in that future world we've created in our imaginings.

This is your magic, your creation towards the future; your future, and the future of everyone you love and everyone they love.

Remember, there's nothing stopping you except agreement that "it can't be done".

I believe women have the vital role in society of putting things in perspective; to guide, to soften the harsh demands of life with her feminine spirit, to get tough when needed, to make things happen that better conditions, no matter what. She does that by believing in herself.

Your health and your beauty are dependent on the decisions you make for yourself now, and the role or roles you choose to assume from this day forward. You have an amazing opportunity to set an example of what we all want to have renewed faith in: that we can be who we really are.

You hold the future in your hands.

Shine my sisters! It's your time to let your inner radiance glow outward to a planet so in need of you.

I wish for you the beautiful life you've always wanted to live. You deserve it.

Make it so.

With my love,

Jeanne

Appendices

Appendix 1

How to Have Beautiful Skin and Get Rid of Wrinkles!

First of all, don't judge your skin. I will be most unhappy with you if you do! Try not to judge it especially first thing in the morning or late at night. Looking in the mirror and saying to your face, "Oh, no! Look at those wrinkles... or those sags... or those blotches... or, or, or!" creates the reality that your skin has those imperfections and makes them more so.

Nature will help your skin return to its natural beauty if you give it a chance.

I procrastinated in writing about what I do for my skin. Then one day my good friend Debbie called me and said; "Jeanne, your skin is the talk of the town! We hate you! (said lovingly of course)." I thought to myself "But... but... but... it's not perfect!"

I then told her some of what I do to handle wrinkles and she said "Jeanne, you've got to let women know!" I've had others say the same but not with the same insistence. Thanks Deb.

Here we go:

CHEMICALS

There are hundreds, if not thousands of harmful chemicals in beauty and body-care products: shampoos, conditioners, moisturizers, cleansers and make-up. You'll look good in the short term using chemical products. But chemicals cause the body to gradually age, including the hair and face. What you do today will show up later as a problem in some other area of health and beauty.

One of the biggest problem-makers is antiperspirants. The major lymph glands are under the arms. The armpits are designed to sweat out toxins. Nature has provided the means to eliminate toxins from the body naturally. If perspiration is inhibited, it stops the lymph glands from doing their job of cleansing. We need to let Nature do her job.

Aluminum is put in most of the antiperspirants on the market. There are wonderful all-natural deodorants without aluminum. One way or another, never, ever use antiperspirants, only deodorants. You can also apply baking soda or a natural light powder to your underarm area.

WHAT IS "ORGANIC"?

There is no government regulation of the word "organic" in the personal-care products industry. Many personal-care products have synthetics in them that are being labeled "natural" and "organic."

Per the Organic Consumers Organization, if you purchase a body care product in a health food store that claims to be organic but does not have the USDA certified organic symbol, you have no way of knowing how much organic content that product actually has. Look for the organic symbol on the label.

HOW DOES ONE REVERSE THE AGING PROCESS OF THE FACE?

First, through using pure products with no toxic chemicals, second by following the correct diet and third, by applying the procedures you're about to learn.

Here's how to prevent and help get rid of wrinkles:

1. Water. Drink half your body weight in water, four to six ounces every half hour until the total amount is consumed. Water is the most important element for the skin and helps prevent and eliminate wrinkles.

2. Get a natural hydrator if you live in a dry environment. A great product is one where the main ingredient is Na-PCA. It pulls water from the air to hydrate your skin. Spray it on your face, let it absorb and then apply a small amount of chemical-free moisturizer or oil before putting on makeup.

3. Aloe Vera gel is also helpful in getting rid of wrinkles and healing the skin. It can be incorporated into your regimen by applying it once or twice a week to the whole face. Let it absorb into your skin and then apply a little oil for moisturizing.

4. Oils. The best oils to use on the face are:

- ❧ Coconut oil. Make sure it is certified organic. It gives a smooth and soft texture to the skin.
- ❧ Apricot kernel oil. This is a great oil to apply all over the body in addition to the face as it is light and absorbs easily.
- ❧ Jojoba oil. It also absorbs beautifully as its inherent makeup is closest to the skins' natural oil.
- ❧ Avocado oil. It makes the skin feel like satin.
- ❧ Olive oil. It's wonderful for skin that is especially dry.

Alternate the oils to find which one that best works for you according to the condition of your skin.

Cold-pressing is the only National Organic Program approved process for the extraction of organic oils for very good reasons. Cold-pressing generates very little heat in the pressing. Low heat (less than 110 degrees) is crucial in cold-pressing because it is well-known that higher temperatures destroy vital nutrients and can cause trans-fats to form.

Choose body care products made without synthetics and preservatives. Instead, look for cold-pressed organic jojoba, coconut, apricot, coconut and avocado oils and select organic botanical extracts.

5. Vitamin E oil. Pure, organic vitamin E oil is truly miraculous in eliminating wrinkles. The women who take my advice about vitamin E oil thank me profusely!

Vitamin E is a natural antioxidant. It helps form normal red blood cells, muscle and other tissues. It protects fat in the body's tissues from abnormal breakdown. Experimental evidence shows vitamin E may protect the heart and blood vessels and retard aging. So it's easy to see how vitamin E will not only slow down the aging process of the face, but may actually rebuild the skin.

Here's what you do: After cleansing and moisturizing your face, gently dab organic 100% Vitamin E oil on wrinkled areas: forehead, lips, jowls, "crow's feet", wherever your skin needs it. Pat it in gently before you go to bed. Don't worry about your pillow case getting a little messy. It's worth it!

Vitamin E heals and puffs up wrinkled areas. Do not apply it on top of or below the eyes as you don't want those areas puffy.

It's best to use the pure vitamin E oil that comes in a little glass bottle from the health-food store. Vitamin E oil in capsules works also but open them up first to check for rancidity. The way to test for rancidity is; place a little of the oil in the back of your throat. If it burns, it's rancid. Replace it.

Vitamin E is just the thing for those specific, tough wrinkled areas. Coconut, apricot kernel, jojoba, avocado and olive oil are for the face overall. These, except for vitamin E oil, are fine to use on the eyelids and below the eyes.

6. Para-Amino Benzoic Acid (PABA). It is known for its ability to absorb ultraviolet (UV) light, thus reducing wrinkling of the skin. Whenever I know I'm going to be spending a lot of time in the sun, along with using protective natural make-up, I take the vitamin PABA internally. I've found it helps stop the sun from burning my skin. Some people are allergic to PABA so check with your nutritionist first.

SAGGING OF THE SKIN

A lot of the reason for sagging skin, as in "jowls" is due to lack of high-quality organic protein. The muscles in the face are like the muscles anywhere else in the body. They need protein and they need exercise to build the muscle.

A great product for exercising the facial muscles is called "Facial Flex." While holding it in your mouth, repeatedly tighten your lips and release. Do this for a few minutes until you can feel the muscles around your mouth and cheeks tightening up. It works great.

CLEANSING AND MOISTURIZING PROCEDURE

Before you go to sleep:

a. To remove your mascara safely, first fold a piece of Kleenex and lay it flat under your lower lashes. Take a light oil, apply it to a Q-tip, close your eyes then gently smear the Q-tip on your upper lashes while holding the Kleenex securely under the lower lashes. Stroke the lashes gently with the Q-tip (with closed eyes) so the mascara ends up on the Kleenex. This will remove the mascara on the lower lashes also. This procedure protects the delicate skin underneath the eyes.

b. Wash your hands well and then wash the makeup off your face using a natural, chemical-free cleanser. Wash and rinse with warm water only, never hot. End off with cool to cold water to close the pores.

c. Exfoliate your skin using a facial scrub made of very fine particles. Otherwise it can tear your skin. Baking soda is great to exfoliate with as its particles are very fine. Try it. You'll see how soft, smooth and clean your skin is afterwards.

d. Pat your face and neck dry.

e. Apply hydrating spray if needed.

f. Apply a small amount of coconut, apricot kernel, jojoba or avocado oil or an organic, all-natural moisturizer to your face and neck. I use about a third of a teaspoon. Keep your eyes closed to make sure the oil doesn't seep into your eyes.

g. Pat Vitamin E oil into the wrinkled areas.

h. Go to sleep.

It's up to you if you want to wash your face again in the morning. I never do. I like to let the oils continue to nourish my skin. If your skin is oily in the morning, pat the excess oil off your face with a clean towel before applying makeup.

If your skin has absorbed the oil or moisturizer during the night, you can apply more in the morning.

OILY SKIN

If your skin is oily or has a tendency towards acne, use a white cotton washcloth when cleansing. Each time be sure to use a clean washcloth washed in chemical-free laundry detergent. Make sure the cleanser you use is not too drying as the skin will rebel by producing more oil.

With oily skin, you may be saying to yourself, "I can't use oil on my skin!" First of all, stop using chemical products on your skin. Consume no heated oils (as in fried food, potato chips, etc). Oils that have been heated before you buy them and oils that have been heated during cooking are toxic. They will cause skin to be unnecessarily oily and break out.

Try coconut oil and see how you do with it. If that doesn't work, get a pure, certified-organic face cream. Once your skin returns to normal through refraining from using cooked oils, experiment using other oils on your face such as jojoba or apricot kernel oil.

For many years I've used only organic cold-pressed oils on my face. My skin used to be oily in the "T zone" (the forehead and nose) and it used to break out. Since applying the information you just read, I've had no problems. And believe me, I had them all.

See the "Products" section at www.themodernrapunzel.com for where to obtain wonderful chemical-free body and skin-care products.

Tips for beautiful skin:

- Always remove makeup before going to bed. Apply the cleansing and moisturizing procedure.
- Use only natural chemical-free makeup obtainable from most health food stores.
- Apply a liquid natural body soap to a body brush or glove exfoliator and then wash your body. This activity wakes up the skin, detoxifies and makes it very soft and silky, especially if you apply a light amount of apricot kernel or jojoba oil to your body afterwards.
- Sitting in a sauna for a comfortable period of time cleans the skin like nothing else can. The skin is refreshed, clean and takes on a wonderful glow. It works wonders!
- See the chapter on "Slant Boards: The Most Vital Piece of Equipment You'll Ever Own" for the massage technique that is miraculous in re-charging skin and making one look years younger.
- The use of an electrical massager on the face on low setting increases circulation which helps drain toxins and reduces puffiness.
- Drugs and alcohol rob the skin and body of vital nutrients. Stay away from them, except for required medications.
- Always wear rubber dish gloves while doing the dishes.
- If you have facial habits like chewing on your lip or pulling on your face, cease doing that.

❧ Wear makeup only when you're going out or doing indoor or outdoor work to protect your skin. The skin needs to breathe as much as possible.

SKIN REJUVENATOR

This is done after a thorough cleansing of your face. Take one-third of an avocado, mash it until it's smooth and creamy. Add about ten homeopathic cell salts (available in a health-food store). Let the cell salts melt in the avocado mash and mix again. Apply to your face and let it sit on your skin for half an hour to an hour. This is fantastic in helping nourish and rejuvenate your skin.

THE MOST IMPORTANT FOR THE SKIN IS

❧ No chemical products, just oils and completely pure moisturizers, creams and cleansers
❧ Water
❧ Vitamin E oil for wrinkles
❧ Facial massage while on a slant board
❧ Diet

SUNSCREENS

There are companies that make "organic" sunscreens but many contain synthetic chemicals. However, there are some good sunscreens with beneficial ingredients.

This is how to use them: Apply your moisturizer. Wait ten minutes, and then apply sunscreen. Wait another ten minutes before applying make-up so the sunscreen can set up its barrier.

Mineral makeup is a good sunscreen although it can be too drying for some skin types. Sesame oil is great for tanning and some say is supposed to stop sunburns.

A small amount of sun is healthy because of the vitamin D the sun provides. Early parts of the day and late in the afternoon are the best times to be out in the sun. When venturing out during the hottest time, cover yourself properly with loose-fitting clothing and a big floppy hat.

Here's a link from Dr. Joseph Mercola's website for help with what sunscreens to avoid and which ones are safe: http://articles.mercola.com/sites/articles/archive/2011/06/06/do-you-know-which-sunscreen-products-to-avoid.aspx

MAKEUP

Beware of most lipsticks. A good percentage of them contain lead which is extremely toxic to the body and can cause learning and behavioral problems. A recent study showed that 61% of 33 brand-name lipsticks have lead in them. It also says that the Food and Drug Administration has not set a limit for lead in lipstick.

Many companies promote "natural makeup" while the makeup is filled with age-producing chemical ingredients.

Most health-food stores carry cosmetics. Have them show you an ingredient list and ensure there are no toxins, lead or parabens in any makeup you buy. Parabens are highly dangerous to the whole body. Eliminate them completely.

Because there are generally no preservatives in natural makeup, you'll need to replace them more often. I recommend replacing them once every three months or so. In the long run you're saving money as you're not compromising your health.

Remember, vitamin E oil is an anti-oxidant which is a natural preservative. By adding it to your liquid organic products, they won't spoil as quickly. Some of the liquid products have a shorter shelf life so this is a great solution and you'll never have to buy foundations with paraben preservatives.

SOME FUN IDEAS

A wonderful tip for using liquid foundation:

After I told a friend about vitamin E oil, she made her own discovery. She mixes equal parts of organic liquid foundation and vitamin E oil and then applies the mixture to her face. Her skin has become super-silky, glows and looks much more youthful. Foundation with vitamin E oil gives the same coverage and the skin is getting nourished all day long.

She also used to apply a bronzer after applying foundation but now it's not needed because the glow the vitamin E brings to her skin is far more radiant. After doing this for a few days, she ran into an old friend who didn't recognize her as she is de-aging from this one simple thing!

There's two ways of mixing it: One, make a palette in the morning and mix your makeup with the oil before applying to your face. Or two, take a small amount of foundation, put it in a little screw-top jar, add the oil and stir. The combination can separate slightly so you'll need to re-stir or shake each time you use it.

ACNE

Acne, blackheads and boils are indicators of other conditions. Dr. Ian Shillington, a very well-known Naturopath, says the three major causes of acne are: 1) poor-functioning kidneys, 2) a toxic bowel and 3) the system is too acidic. The majority of the time it's a combination of all three. Dehydration is also a key factor in acne problems.

How is it that acne occurs as a result of these factors? The body uses the skin as a back-up elimination organ if the kidneys and bowels are not operating one hundred percent.

How to handle acne:

a. The system needs to be given more alkaline foods to neutralize the acid condition. One of the best ways to alkalize the body is by eating vegetables, fresh or steamed, and drinking vegetable juices. To speed up the process of alkalizing your body, you can also add a little baking soda or alkaline drops from the health-food store to your drinking water.

b. Get plenty of exercise and take hot and cold showers to move the blood through the system. By doing this you are moving toxins out.

c. Stay away from cooked oils. The only oils acceptable to use in cooking are olive, sesame and coconut oils on *very* low heat.

d. Acidophilus provides good bacteria for the intestines. It has shown to be miraculous in alleviating acne.

Antibiotics cover up the underlying reasons for acne. They destroy the beneficial bacteria in the body. It's wise to take them only when you have to. Talk with your doctor.

  e. Change your pillow case every night so you're not putting bacteria back onto your skin.
  f. Keep your hands away from your face.

Eyes

DARK CIRCLES UNDER THE EYES

Dark circles under the eyes are usually an indicator of liver and/or kidney problems. When you clean out those organs, the circles diminish or go away completely. It starts with cleaning out the intestines first. Then the cleansing of the liver and kidneys is much easier and more efficient.

Dark circles are sometimes inherited. Dark circles can also come from allergies, not enough sleep or a shadow being cast from the bone under the eye.

PUFFY EYES

If your eyes are puffy in the morning it could be from one of the following:

  a. Dust mites in your pillow case. Obtain a dust-mite protective case and then put a regular pillow case over that.
  b. Eating before you go to bed or late at night, especially fried food (as in fried chicken or French Fries) or carbohydrates with salt (as in crackers) and refined wheat products (as in pasta and white bread) will show up on your eyes and face the next day.
  c. Not drinking your quota of water the previous day.
  d. Chemical products used on the eyes. The best thing to use for the skin under the eye and on the eyelid is a light application of coconut, jojoba, apricot kernel, avocado oil or another all-natural product.

HOW TO HELP REDUCE PUFFY EYES

1. Warm, moist tea bags, (mostly chamomile) cucumber or potato slices placed over the eyes will reduce puffiness.
2. A super-thin layer of whipped egg whites under the eyes. It also helps nourish the area.
3. Never rub your under-eye area with anything, especially facial tissue.
4. Taking a sauna helps decrease puffy eyes.

How to Whiten Your Teeth Naturally!

My friend Peggy told me of a wonderful way to naturally whiten teeth. Get some cold-pressed organic safflower, sesame or coconut oil. Put one tablespoon of one of the oils in your mouth. Suck the oil in, out and through your teeth. (Make sure you don't swallow any of the oil.) Do this for about ten minutes, spit it out and then thoroughly rinse your mouth with 3% Hydrogen Peroxide Solution and spit that out. This procedure not only whitens your teeth but pulls toxins from the lymphatic system.

You may already know some of the tips here but I hope you've learned some others and will apply them. If you do, watch your "age" go down, down, down!

Let's look at the cost of a chemical peel or face lift versus the simple techniques described here. The average surgeon's fee for a face lift is $9,500, the anesthesiologist fee is $6,000, the facility fee is $1,200 and the hospital fee $1,700. Let's see, what does that come to? $18,400. That's the average.

That practically buys enough organic oils for a small city!

Have lots of fun with your new techniques!

Appendix 2

Standard Shampooing Procedure

USING A CLARIFYING SHAMPOO WHEN THERE'S HEAVY CHEMICAL BUILD-UP

a. To shampoo correctly using this procedure, combine clarifying shampoo and regular chemical-free shampoo, half of each, onto the palms of your hands, lather and then apply. Do not pour any shampoo directly onto your scalp.

b. Gently scrub your scalp for less than a minute with the shampoo mixture. Yes, I said just the scalp, not your whole head of hair.

c. After shampooing the scalp, pull the shampoo through the hair once or twice. Never, ever scrub the hair itself.

d. Rinse immediately and thoroughly. Reminder: Ensure that you rinse with medium-low to low water pressure and lukewarm water temperature only. Medium-low water pressure and medium-low water temperature are very key to the health of your hair.

e. Condition your hair, not your scalp, with a chemical-free conditioner. Leave the conditioner in until it's had a chance to do its job of softening your hair, which can take as long as five minutes. You can wash the rest of your body during that time.

f. Rinse your hair again for 20-30 seconds with slightly warm water. Then gradually make the water cooler and cooler until it's as cold as you can comfortably handle. This closes the cuticle and provides circulation to the scalp. The whole rinsing procedure takes less than a minute.

g. With your head upside-down, squeeze the excess water in your hair into a towel and then wrap your hair in the towel for a couple minutes before combing. Do not ever use friction on your hair or scalp. Be gentle.

h. Using a wide-toothed comb, gently comb your hair out starting from the bottom and work up. Work the tangles out slowly not allowing your hair to snap. If tangles don't come out easily, apply a dime to a quarter-sized amount (the amount depending on whether your hair is long or short) of chemical-free, leave-in conditioner onto one palm, distribute the conditioner evenly on both hands and then gently stroke the tangled parts of your hair with your "conditioned" hands (never the scalp). You might need to squeeze the conditioner into any especially tangled spots with your hands. Resume gentle combing from the bottom. The comb should now glide through the hair. Leave the conditioner in. Do not rinse out.

i. If possible, let your hair dry naturally.

USING YOUR OWN HOME-MADE CLARIFIER

Repeat the full instructions above for shampooing and conditioning but now you will be using a home-made clarifier instead of a clarifying shampoo. The home-made clarifier consists of a vinegar rinse. Clarifying shampoo is used only when there's heavy chemical build-up. A vinegar rinse is applied per the schedule as outlined below.

1. Have a 16-ounce plastic cup in your shower.
2. Have a quart of organic Apple Cider Vinegar (Braggs is the best) accessible in your bathroom.
3. Before you get into the shower, put 3 tablespoons of vinegar in the plastic cup and add warm water to the top.
4. Take this mixture into the shower with you.
5. After you've shampooed your hair and before you condition it, take the vinegar rinse and starting at the crown of your head, let it run down and over your whole scalp and hair.
6. Rinse immediately.
7. Apply conditioner.
8. Rinse.

Vinegar rinse removes shampoo residue from the hair. This is important as residue from shampoo is drying to the hair.

The schedule is:

1. Wash your hair mixing half clarifying shampoo and half regular shampoo together once every two weeks, or more as necessary if there's heavy build-up.

2. Depending on how often you shampoo your hair, the general rule is to use the vinegar rinse every other time you wash your hair except when you need to use the clarifying shampoo. I've found that using the vinegar rinse every time I wash my hair is too drying.

Appendix 3: Charts

These charts are not a substitute for the full information contained in the body of this book. When you find you need more detailed understanding and instructions, please refer back to the relevant sections.

The first procedure you will come to in this charts section is "Standard Procedures for Hair in All Conditions". This is the unvarying procedure to be followed for optimum hair growth for hair in *all* conditions. It is very important you follow this no matter the current condition of your hair. You will need to refer back to this over and over again until the procedures become second nature.

Then you will find the category relating to the specific condition of your hair. This gives you the procedures to be implemented for your category *in addition* to the Standard Procedures.

Please look at the three categories below to determine which additional chart applies to your situation:

CATEGORY 1: "NEEDS A LITTLE HELP"

This is additional procedure for hair that is starting to show some signs of damage (dry and/or brittle), not thick enough, is not growing to your satisfaction and has little to no luster.

CATEGORY 2: "I'M STARTING TO GET WORRIED"

This is additional procedure for hair that not only has signs of damage, is not growing and has lack of luster; but is thinning. Concern has set in.

CATEGORY 3: "YIKES! MY HAIR, WHAT THERE IS LEFT OF IT, IS A DISASTER!"

This is additional procedure for hair that is badly damaged and thinning out of control.

These charts make it easy for you to see "at-a-glance" what procedures and tools are needed to turn your situation around.

As an added note, it is beneficial to take a look at the procedures in the other two categories. In other words, if your hair is in the "Needs a little help" category, you can always refer to the other two categories which ensure even greater results.

Standard Procedures for Hair in All Conditions

3-STEP MAGIC OVERNIGHT HAIR BEAUTIFICATION

This procedure helps restore strength and elasticity to your hair immediately.

1. Use a *chlorine shower filter* while washing your hair.
2. Use a *gentle, non-toxic clarifying shampoo* to remove toxic build-up.
3. To restore elasticity and thickness, *use oils.* This procedure is fully explained in Chapter One.

SPLIT ENDS

Cut them all off.

USE OF HAIR PRODUCTS

Use only chemical-free hair care products.

SHAMPOOING AND CONDITIONING

See the two procedures at the beginning of this section: 1) shampooing with a clarifying shampoo and 2) using your own home-made clarifier.

Rotate your shampoos and conditioners. Have three to four chemical-free shampoos and conditioners on hand at all times.

Keep your *water pressure low to medium-low and keep the water temperature lukewarm* while shampooing and rinsing your hair. For the final rinse, start with lukewarm water then gradually make the water cool and then cold.

Gently scrub only the scalp, then pull the shampoo through to the ends. Never scrub the hair itself with shampoo.

Use conditioner on your hair only, never the scalp.

If possible, *let your hair dry naturally.*

STYLING

To prevent burning, *keep the curling and/or flat iron moving and on medium to medium-low heat* while you're styling. If your hair is especially damaged, use wraps obtained from a beauty supply store to prevent heat from damaging your hair.

Never allow hairspray to come in contact with your scalp. Use a pump spray, not aerosol.

Do not use any products on your scalp except shampoo and the oils as directed in the section on scalp massage.

If your hair is thinning where you part it, switch the part to the other side.

BRUSHING, COMBING AND MASSAGE

Use a wide-toothed comb on wet hair, never a brush. Comb from the bottom up, gently working out tangles as you go.

Brush your hair <u>only</u> when it's dry. Use a brush that has widely-spaced bristles with rounded ends or a boars bristle brush.

Brush hair daily for circulation. Brush upside-down starting at the nape of the neck.

Use a massager on your scalp at least three times a week for thirty seconds to a minute, using no oil.

HAIR COLOR AND PERMANENTS

Before coloring or perming your hair, do the elasticity test to see if your hair is strong enough to withstand the chemicals.

Do not perm <u>and</u> color your hair. Having both procedures done to your hair is a sure route to disaster for hair in any condition.

USE OF OILS TO HELP RESTORE ELASTICITY AND STRENGTH

See Step 3 of the Magic Overnight Hair Beautification Procedure for the procedure on how, when and what oils to apply to your hair.

SLANT BOARD

A slant board is essential to new hair growth. Massage the scalp while lying on a slant board. See the full scalp-massage procedure in the section on slant boards.

Diet and Health Routines

NUTRITION AND DIET

Get *high-quality protein* in your diet in the right amount.
See "The Rules" on what to eat.
See the "On-Going Diet Regimen".
Vegetable juicing
Omega 3, 6, 9 (Essential Fatty Acids)

VITAMINS AND MINERALS

Take a good source of *whole, live vitamins* in balance – vitamins A, B, C, D and E. Vitamin B is especially important for hair growth. Ensure you take the other vitamins and minerals needed to balance the B's.

Take calcium, magnesium, potassium, sodium and trace minerals.

Take PABA and Panothenic Acid as directed by your natural health-care practitioner.

HORMONES

Eat hormone and antibiotic-free, organic meats only.

Get your *hormones tested* by a competent health-care practitioner if you feel they might be out of balance.

SLEEP

Get the amount of sleep you need to be fully rested.

WATER

Divide your body weight by two. *Drink that total amount of water in ounces,* 4-6 ounces at a time every half hour.

Drink distilled water (in glass bottles or obtain your own distiller) and spring water from a natural spring. If your pH level is on the acidic side, add *baking soda* to your water per the instructions in the chapter on water.

EXERCISE

Exercise for a half an hour to an hour every day. See the procedure on how to exercise.

TOXINS

Stay away from barbecued, fried and processed foods, sugar, Coca-Cola, soft drinks (unless from the health-food store), caffeine, MSG, microwave ovens and artificial sweeteners.

If you don't have a filter on your sink, *wear gloves while doing dishes and washing vegetables.*

Eliminate *toxic cleaning products*, laundry detergent and fabric softeners from your home and office.

STRESS

See Chapter Thirteen, "The Factors of Stress and Hair Loss" and Section Two, "You: The Whole Woman." Find the chapter that relates to your life now and refer back to it as often as needed until you have that area of your life improved or mastered, then onto to the next if there is more than one area you need help with.

BASIC AND ESSENTIAL STANDARD ITEMS FOR ALL CATEGORIES:

- Chlorine filter for your shower
- Chemical-free clarifying shampoo, regular shampoos, conditioners, hair spray, hair gel
- A wide-toothed comb
- Brush that has widely-spaced bristles and rounded rubber ends
- Live Vitamins
- Minerals
- Slant Board
- Juicer

See the "Products" section at www.themodernrapunzel.com for where to obtain them.

⁓

Category 1: "Needs a Little Help"

This is additional procedure for hair that is starting to show some signs of damage (dry and/or brittle), not thick enough, is not growing to your satisfaction and has little to no luster.

SPLIT ENDS

To prevent dry ends from splitting, combine jojoba and vitamin E oil and saturate the ends with this mixture. Leave on for at least an hour and wash out gently.

USE OF OILS ON THE HAIR AND SCALP TO HELP RESTORE ELASTICITY AND STRENGTH TO THE HAIR

See Step 3 of the Magic Overnight Hair Beautification Procedure for the procedure on how, when and what oils to apply.

HAIR COLOR AND PERMANENTS

If your hair is falling out or thin, do not perm your hair. Get a good haircut to suit your face until your hair is in shape to be permed.

If you need to color your hair, try to find a salon that uses organic hair color or go to the health-food store and find a color that works for you.

Before you perm or color, do the elasticity test.

CHIROPRACTIC ADJUSTMENTS as needed.

TO ELIMINATE JUNK FOOD CRAVINGS. See "For Your Hair's Sake"

BASIC AND ESSENTIAL ITEMS TO HAVE:

❧ Chlorine filter for your shower

- Chemical-free clarifying shampoo, regular shampoos, conditioners, hair spray, hair gel
- A wide-toothed comb
- Brush that has widely-spaced bristles and rounded rubber ends
- Live Vitamins
- Minerals
- Slant Board
- Juicer

Here are the items to obtain for this category in addition to the basic and essential items listed above.

- Oils: jojoba oil is the first and foremost oil to have on hand. Extra virgin olive oil, apricot kernel oil and avocado oil are optional, but are a very good idea as the oils will work differently at different times according to the condition of your hair. They are available from your health-food store.
- Electric massager for your scalp.

See the "Products" section at www.themodernrapunzel.com for where to obtain them.

Category 2: "I'm Starting to Get Worried"

This is additional procedure for hair that not only has signs of damage, is not growing and has lack of luster; but is thinning. Concern has set in.

SPLIT ENDS

To prevent dry ends from splitting, combine jojoba and vitamin E oil and saturate the ends with this mixture. Leave on for at least an hour and wash out gently.

If you're a swimmer, use a swim cap and saturate your hair and scalp with a thick oil, like olive oil. Concentrate the oil on the front hairline. Much better yet, swim in an ocean, lake or chlorine-free pool.

SHAMPOOING AND CONDITIONING

Wash your hair every two to four days, not every day.
   Never wash your hair where it becomes squeaky clean.
   Try to use only non oil-based shampoos and conditioners with the exception of natural shampoos designed to handle hair loss.
   Put shampoo on your hands first, lather and then apply. Do not pour the shampoo directly onto your scalp.
   Do not use friction with a towel while drying your hair. Instead, squeeze out the excess water and then use the towel as a turban.

HAIR COLOR AND PERMANENTS

If your hair is falling out or thin, do not perm your hair. Get a good haircut to suit your face until your hair is in shape to be permed.
   If you need to color your hair, try to find a salon that uses organic hair color or go to the health food store and find a color that works for your hair.
   Before you perm or color, do the elasticity test.

USE OF OILS ON THE HAIR AND SCALP TO HELP RESTORE ELASTICITY AND STRENGTH TO THE HAIR

See Step Three of Magic Overnight Hair Beautification.
   If your scalp is oily, do not use oils on your scalp. Instead, massage your scalp using the massage procedures laid out in the book.

Eliminate cooked oils and fatty animal products.

Very lightly coat the outside top layer of your hair, not the scalp with *coconut or apricot kernel oil* to handle the frizzies.

USE OF A SLANT BOARD

A slant board is essential to new hair growth. It is ideal to massage the scalp while laying on a slant board. See the procedure in the section on slant boards.

To de-congest the follicles, massage scalp with jojoba or castor oil while on a slant board. See the full scalp massage procedure in the section on slant boards.

HAIR RESTRAINTS

Limit or eliminate restraints (barrettes, bobby pins, wigs, etc.)

If you have to wear hats, helmets or headbands, ensure you remove them often as they make the scalp hold oil and perspiration which clog the follicles.

Do not do hair weaving, wear wigs or have hair extensions put in your hair. Instead implement the procedures in this book.

CHIROPRACTIC ADJUSTMENTS as needed.

TOXINS

Rid your body of toxins. This is a major contributing factor to hair loss and overall health and well-being. See the section on detoxification.

Gradually implement vegetable juices and/or a nutritious greens supplement into your diet.

Eliminate toxic household cleaning products, laundry detergent and fabric softeners from your home and office.

TO ELIMINATE JUNK FOOD CRAVINGS see "For Your Hair's Sake"

MISCELLANEOUS

Do not consume cooked oils and fatty animal products except for coconut, olive and sesame oils used at low temperature.

Have your thyroid and adrenal function checked.

If there is a *scalp infection* and it doesn't handle easily or if you're on medicines that you think may be affecting your hair, see a competent health-care practitioner.

Instead of worrying, envision your hair the way you want it to look. In doing this you will feel empowered to continue. Your health, body and hair will respond.

BASIC AND ESSENTIAL ITEMS TO HAVE:

- Chlorine filter for your shower
- Chemical-free clarifying shampoo, regular shampoos, conditioners, hair spray, hair gel
- A wide toothed comb
- Brush that has widely-spaced bristles and rounded rubber ends
- Live Vitamins
- Minerals
- Slant Board
- Juicer

Here are the items to obtain for this category in addition to the basic and essential items:

- Oils: jojoba oil is the first and foremost oil to have on hand. Extra virgin olive oil, apricot kernel oil and avocado oil are optional, but are a very good idea as the oils will work differently at different times according to the condition of your hair. These are available at your health-food store.
- Electric massager for your scalp
- Follicle de-tox product
- Powdered green product
- Hormones (have them tested)
- Intestinal cleansing product
- Chemical-free cleaning and household products
- Chemical-free skin and body products
- Foot bath and/or foot pads
- Liquid zeolite

See the "Products" section at www.themodernrapunzel.com for where to obtain them.

Category 3:
"Yikes! My Hair, What There Is Left Of It, Is a Disaster!"

This is additional procedure for hair that is badly damaged and is thinning out of control.

SPLIT ENDS

To prevent dry ends from splitting, combine jojoba and vitamin E oil and saturate the ends with this mixture. Leave on for at least an hour and wash out gently.

If you're a swimmer, use a swim cap and saturate your hair and scalp with a thick oil, like olive oil. Do this so the chlorine from the water doesn't absorb into your hair. Concentrate the oil on the front hairline. Much better yet, swim in an ocean or lake.

SHAMPOOING AND CONDITIONING

Wash your hair every two to four days, not every day.
Never wash your hair to the point where it becomes squeaky clean.
Try to use only non oil-based shampoos and conditioners with the exception of natural shampoos designed to handle hair loss.
Put shampoo on your hands first, lather and then apply. Do not pour the shampoo directly onto your scalp.
Do not use friction with a towel while drying your hair. Instead, squeeze out the excess water and then use the towel as a turban.

USE OF OILS ON THE HAIR AND SCALP TO HELP RESTORE ELASTICITY AND STRENGTH TO THE HAIR

See Step Three of the Magic Overnight Hair Beautification Procedure.

If your scalp is oily, do not use oils on your scalp. Instead, massage your scalp using the massage procedures as laid out in the book.

Eliminate cooked oils and fatty animal products.

Very lightly coat the top layer of your hair with *coconut oil* to handle the frizzies.

USE OF A SLANT BOARD

A slant board is essential to new hair growth. It is ideal to massage the scalp while laying on a slant board. See the massage procedure in the section on slant boards.

To de-congest the follicles, massage scalp with jojoba or castor oil while on a slant board. See the full scalp massage procedure in the section on slant boards.

HAIR COLOR AND PERMANENTS

If your hair is falling out or thin, do not perm your hair. Get a good haircut to suit your face until your hair is in shape to be permed.

If you need to color your hair, try to find a salon that uses organic hair color or go to the health food store and find a color that works for your hair.

Before you perm or color, do the elasticity test.

HAIR RESTRAINTS

Limit or eliminate restraints (barrettes, bobby pins, wigs, etc.)

If you have to wear hats, helmets or headbands, ensure you remove them often as they make the scalp hold oil and perspiration which clog the follicles.

Do not do hair weaving, wear wigs or have hair extensions put in your hair. Instead follow the procedures in this book.

CHIROPRACTIC ADJUSTMENTS as needed.

TOXINS

Rid your body of toxins. This is a major contributing factor in hair loss and overall health and well-being. See the section on detoxification.

Gradually implement vegetable juices and a nutritious greens supplement into your diet. This is essential for you.

Eliminate toxic household cleaning products, laundry detergent and fabric softeners from your home and office.

TO ELIMINATE JUNK FOOD CRAVINGS see "For Your Hair's Sake".

MISCELLANEOUS

Do not consume cooked oils and fatty animal products except for coconut, olive and sesame oils used at very low temperature.

Have your thyroid and adrenal function checked.

If there is a *scalp infection* and it doesn't handle easily or if you're on medicines that you think may be affecting your hair, see a competent health-care practitioner.

Instead of worrying, envision your hair the way you want it to look. In doing this you will feel empowered to continue. Your health, body and hair will respond.

BASIC AND ESSENTIAL ITEMS TO HAVE:

- Chlorine filter for your shower
- Chemical-free clarifying shampoo, regular shampoos, conditioners, hair spray, hair gel
- A wide-toothed comb
- Brush that has widely-spaced bristles and rounded rubber ends
- Live Vitamins
- Minerals
- Slant Board
- Juicer

Here are the items to obtain for this category in addition to the basic and essential items:

- Oils: jojoba oil is the first and foremost oil to have on hand. Extra virgin olive oil, apricot kernel oil and avocado oil are optional, but are a very good idea as the oils will work differently at different times according to the condition of your hair. Available from your health-food store.

- Electric massager for your scalp
- Follicle de-tox product
- Powdered green product
- Hormones (have them tested)
- Intestinal cleansing product
- Intestinal, liver and kidney cleanse
- Chemical-free cleaning products
- Chemical-free skin and body products
- Foot bath and/or foot pads
- Liquid zeolite

See the "Products" section at www.themodernrapunzel.com for where to obtain them.

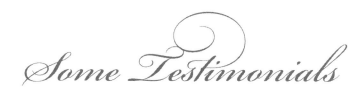

Some Testimonials

"Someone recommended your book and I jumped at the chance to buy a copy. I read it and said, "Finally, something easy enough for me to be able to do!" I can now not only tell a difference in the feel of my hair but in the thickness. It's growing better and faster than it has ever done before. I love it!!! I can't say enough good things about you and your book. Thank you!!!" ⁓ DA

"I have to tell you - I washed my hair this morning and not one hair came out!! Is that awesome, or what?! And my husband notices my hair looks more vibrant!" ⁓ LL

"After reading your book and putting in several of the points, my hair has grown about 5 inches and is not frizzy. No one tells me to cut my hair any-more. And now I even will look in the mirror every so often, when before this change it was not worth looking in the mirror!!" ⁓ CH

"Jeanne, you are my Hairy Godmother!

"After reading and applying your methods on how to grow hair, I am astonished at the results I'm getting after just three weeks! I've always had thin, limp hair that won't grow past my shoulders no matter what I do. I've tried every product on the market from expensive hair thickeners to conditioners and have even gone to drastic measures and had hair exten-sions. But in just three weeks I've seen miracles!

"The combination of these simple and inexpensive remedies has been unbelievable and has already made a drastic difference in the texture of my hair! You might not believe me, but in just three weeks the new growth is at least four times thicker! My new hair is not limp or lifeless either! It is wavy and lush!

"Okay, I'm going to keep gushing here because I also want to thank you for the skin care advice. I have T-zone oily skin and was never able to use moisturizers on my face because my skin would break out. Now with your procedures not only has my skin not broken out once, but the fine wrinkles around my eyes and on my forehead have almost entirely disappeared. This is just in three weeks. If I keep going with this I'm going to look 20 years old again!" ⌒ KR, Author

"My hair is so lustrous and shiny...I get so many comments on it now. People say I have beautiful hair! I had two people tell me that my hair was absolutely stunning! Can you believe it? Me, the girl who always felt like the ugliest woman in the room because of my horrible hair! I never have bad hair days. Ever.

"My hair is always beautiful now and I am no longer introverted on it. This coming from a woman who didn't live a day of her life not being introverted on her hair. I'm doing really well thanks to your book!" ⌒ MS

"The day after I applied the first treatment, I already had an appointment with my hairdresser. She could not believe the difference in the dryness gone from my hair. She was simply amazed!! She asked me what I was using and I told her, she couldn't believe it! I am trying all of the steps eventually Jeanne, and I think that you are wonderful to help so many women with their problems with their hair! You are certainly right when you say that hair is a Woman's Crowning glory! All the Best Jeanne. You are an incredible woman." ⌒ Fondly, MM

"I coated the top of my head (which is where things are REAL thin) with the product you recommend and in one treatment only, it looks like I have double the thickness. Amazing! Thank you so much - I have hope again." ⌒ EV

"This book has been the best thing I have found. I love the fact that you mention products by name and brands so that I don't have to guess or research for the products. Thank you for sharing your knowledge and experiences through your book. Your book has opened a whole new world of beauty aids and a healthy lifestyle. Thank you so much for sharing your story. I think you are great and you have made a difference in my life." ⌒ Gratefully, EG

"This book is in truth a multi-layered gift of how to best take care of myself and achieve the most aesthetic me I can be, the way I want, naturally. Although for years I have already used many principles of natural health,

I was pleasantly surprised at the many dimensions of application in this book. Jeanne provides answers and inspiration for hair and much more. It is a comprehensive guide to the seriously vain but natural woman." ⁓ PK

"Your procedures for the skin work fabulously! The skin's much more alive, smooth and rosy -like a baby's :). It's really uplifting. The hair is doing very well also; and this just after a few days - with not even all the points you make being applied! It's thicker, very smooth and soft like silk.

"I'm as good as done with the book. What I really liked about it so far, though, was the part about attitude and beauty. That really got me to change my point of view. See, I did all these different things just for a healthy body before - and I studied quite a bit on these issues -I did all these things mainly with only the body, its health in mind, you know.

"I basically forgot that I'm a source of beauty and beauty itself that creates beauty. And you really helped me to change this. Thank you!!! You're a treasure. For me, this was really the best and most valuable part.

"I'm so grateful that you inform about all these technicalities and procedures too. Hair, skin, a working this or that are, however, just consequences of being and radiating beauty. Women are indeed the angels of beauty and joy. You're so right." ⁓ JA

Praise for
The Modern Rapunzel

"I just loved this book. I initially read it to find out how to achieve beautiful, thick hair and found amazingly easy and doable secrets from which I've had great results. The information is straightforward and simple. In addition, it's a great read. Jeanne Powers is funny and inspiring and this book offers so much more than I had imagined. Though it starts being all about a woman's crowning glory it reveals a plethora of knowledge and information one needs to live a happier, more successful and fulfilling life. Her book is brimming with "ah-ha" moments and I recommend it highly!" ∼ MA

"You've got to read this wonderful new book by Jeanne Powers! Finally - a gal who "Walks the Talk". It's not just a treatise on "looking" beautiful, it is the definitive instruction manual on "being" beautiful. Everyone of us is beauty, and Ms. Powers shows one and all how to realize it with complete certainty." ∼ Dr. Ian Shillington

"Magnificent, inspirational, delightful and fun! Forgotten words and practices from wise women of our past brought forward by a wise woman of today. May these words and values never die!" ∼ PC, Nutritionist

"I loved this book.

   "Jeanne is a great story teller, has obvious certainty and conviction about what she writes about, and you really get to know her through this book. I was particularly impressed by the last section of her book, *You: The Whole Woman*. This is the 'in section: truly insightful, inspirational and informational chapters which present Jeanne's philosophy and personal viewpoints that apply to anyone, of any age, that provides a beautiful reality about the factors of aging. Her writing style makes the book effortless to read, easy to follow, and has a clarity of communication that is very impressive.

   I promise you, you will come away with new realities that will inspire you." ∼ BP, author, educator, producer

7369901R00143

Made in the USA
San Bernardino, CA
02 January 2014